STUDENT WORKBOOK TO ACCOMPANY

DENTAL HYGIENE

Applications to Clinical Practice

Tammy R. Sanderson, RDH, MSDH
Assistant Professor
Department of Dental Hygiene
Idaho State University
Pocatello, ID

Rachel Henry, RDH, MS
Assistant Professor
Dental Hygiene Graduate Program Director
Ohio State College of Dentistry, Division of Dental Hygiene
Columbus, OH

Maria Perno Goldie, RDH, BA, MS
Past President, International Federation of Dental Hygienists
Past President, American Dental Hygienists Association
Owner, Seminars for Women's Health and Sex-Based Medicine
Editorial Director, RDH eVillage Focus
Co-founder, International Dental Hygiene Educator's Forum
San Carlos, CA

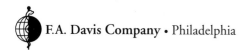 F.A. Davis Company • Philadelphia

F. A. Davis Company
1915 Arch Street
Philadelphia, PA 19103
www.fadavis.com

Copyright © 2016 by F. A. Davis Company

Printed in the United States of America

Last digit indicates print number: 10 9 8 7 6 5 4 3 2 1

Publisher: Quincy McDonald
Director of Content Development: George W. Lang
Developmental Editor: Patricia Gillivan
Art and Design Manager: Carolyn O'Brien

ISBN: 978-0-8036-2569-3

Reviewers

Joanna Allaire, RDH, MDH
Periodontics and Dental Hygiene
The University of Texas School of Dentistry
Houston, TX

Jordan Rae Anderson, RDH, BS, MDH
Dental Hygiene
University of Louisiana Monroe
Monroe, LA

Sandra N. Beebe, RDH, PhD
School Allied Health, ASA
Southern Illinois University Carbondale
Carbondale, IL

Dawn Conley, RDH, MEd
Dental Department
Camden County College
Blackwood, NJ

Shelly M. Costley, RDH, MEd
Dental Hygiene
Weber State University
Ogden, UT

Patricia D. Guenther, RDH, MA
Allied Health & Human Service
Lansing Community College
Lansing, MI

Harold A. Henson, RDH, PhD
Periodontics and Dental Hygiene
The University of Texas School of Dentistry at
Houston
Houston, TX

Kathleen Hodges, RDH, MS
Department of Dental Hygiene, Office of Medical and
Oral Health
Idaho State University
Pocatello, ID

Jacquelyne L. Mack, RDH, MS, MPA
Dental Programs
Florida State College at Jacksonville
Jacksonville, FL

Paula Malcomson, BA, BEd
Dental Programs
Fanshawe College
London, Ontario, Canada

Frances McConaughy, MS, RDH
Dental Hygiene
Weber State University
Ogden, UT

Kristine B. Morrow, BSDH, MHA
School of Dental Hygiene
Old Dominion University
Norfolk, VA

Jo Ann Nyquist, BSDH, MA, EDS
Dental Hygiene
Wayne County Community College District
Detroit, MI

Amanda Richardson, BS, RDH, MDH
Dental Hygiene
University of Louisiana at Monroe
Monroe, LA

Leah W. Rising, BS, MS
Dental Program
Gulf State College
Panama City, FL

Kelly Turner, BA, RDH
Health Sciences: Dental Programs
Fanshawe College
London, Ontario, Canada

Contents

Part I

Introduction to Dental Hygiene

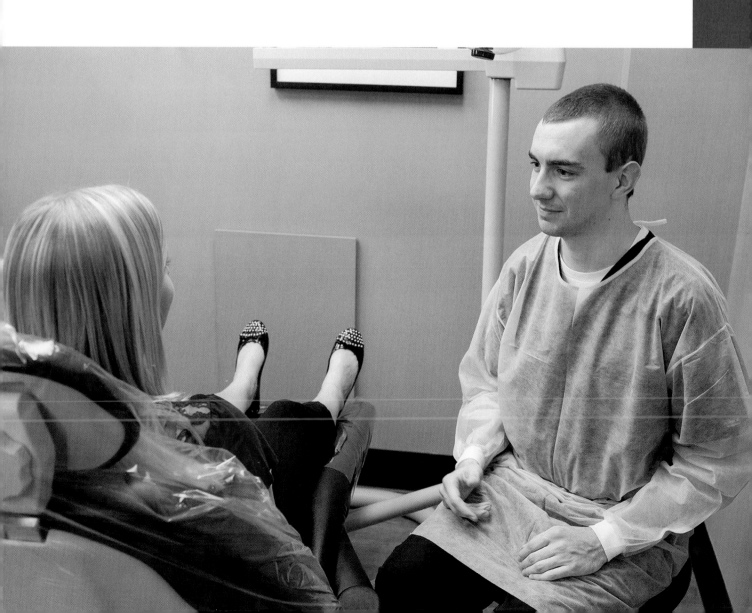

Chapter 1 | Dental Hygiene as a Profession

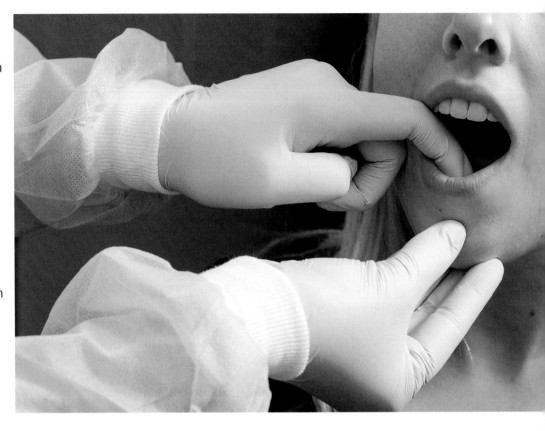

LEARNING OBJECTIVES

After reading this chapter, the student should be able to:

1.1 Define the term *dental hygienist.*
1.2 Describe the history and evolution of dental hygiene practice.
1.3 Describe the roles of the dental hygienist.
1.4 List and explain the dental hygiene process of care.
1.5 Summarize the standards of care for dental hygiene.
1.6 Explain the importance of dental hygiene professional organizations.

KEY CONCEPTS

• A registered dental hygienist (RDH) is a licensed oral health-care
  professional who specializes in preventive oral health.
• Evidence-based decision-making is the foundation of dental hygiene
  education, practice, and research.
• The American Dental Hygienists' Association (ADHA) is the professional
  organization that represents dental hygienists in the United States.
• Dental hygienists are graduates of accredited dental hygiene education
  programs in colleges and universities, and must take a written national board
  examination and a clinical examination before they are licensed to practice.

• The profession of dental hygiene must embrace change, focus on growth and development, and plan for its future, as well as the future oral health needs of the public.

RELEVANCE TO CLINICAL PRACTICE

Entering into a career in dental hygiene is more than just taking a new job. Dental hygiene is a rewarding profession and career choice. **Dental hygienists** are essential members of the dental team and interdisciplinary health-care teams. The profession of dental hygiene began as a **public health** profession and has since evolved into a discipline that continues to grow. The potential for dental hygienists who are clinically trained and have expanded their education is great.

The profession of dental hygiene is more than 100 years old. It is essential that dental hygienists be aware of the profession's history and are part of its future.

The Basics

1. Choose the incorrect phrase as related to the dental hygienist.
   A. Is a licensed preventative oral health professional
   B. Works in a variety of settings
   C. Each state defines the licensure requirements for the dental hygienist
   D. All states require the dental hygienist to have graduated from an accredited dental hygiene program

2. All of the following statements are correct regarding the preventative dental hygiene movement *except* for one. Which one is the *exception?*
   A. The movement began in Cleveland, Ohio.
   B. It was started by the Oral Hygiene Committee of the National Dental Association.
   C. It began as a publicly funded program in hospitals.
   D. It began as a publicly funded program in schools.

3. The dental hygiene scope of practice is determined by:
   A. Individual states
   B. Federal government
   C. Dental hygiene associations
   D. Colleges/Universities

4. Identify the *incorrect* statement.
   A. The ADHA is a professional organization.
   B. Participation by dental hygienists in the ADHA is mandatory.
   C. Membership in the ADHA offers dental hygiene opportunities for professional development.
   D. The ADHA offers resources related to evidence-based clinical recommendations.

5. All of the following statements are true of the first dental hygiene program *except* for one. Which one is the *exception?*
   A. The program was initiated by Dr. Alfred C. Fones.
   B. The program started in Bridgeport, Connecticut.
   C. Dental hygienists were taught to remove plaque biofilm and calculus deposits.
   D. The program started as a private-practice model.

6. The association that serves to unite dental hygiene associations is the:
   A. International Federation of Dental Hygienists (IFDH)
   B. National Dental Hygienists' Association (NDHA)
   C. American Dental Hygienists' Association (ADHA)

7. List the six standards of care for dental hygiene.

   1) _____
   _____

   2) _____
   _____

   3) _____
   _____

   4) _____
   _____

   5) _____
   _____

   6) _____
   _____

Learning Activities

1. Identify and describe the roles of the dental hygienist.

_____
_____
_____
_____
_____
_____
_____
_____
_____
_____
_____
_____
_____
_____
_____
_____
_____
_____
_____
_____

2. Explain the dental hygiene process of care.

_____

_____

_____

_____

_____

_____

_____

_____

_____

_____

_____

_____

_____

_____

_____

_____

_____

_____

_____

Chapter 2 | Legal and Ethical Considerations

KEY TERMS

autonomy
beneficence
confidentiality
civil law
criminal law
ethical decision-making
fiduciary
justice
nonmaleficence
societal trust
veracity

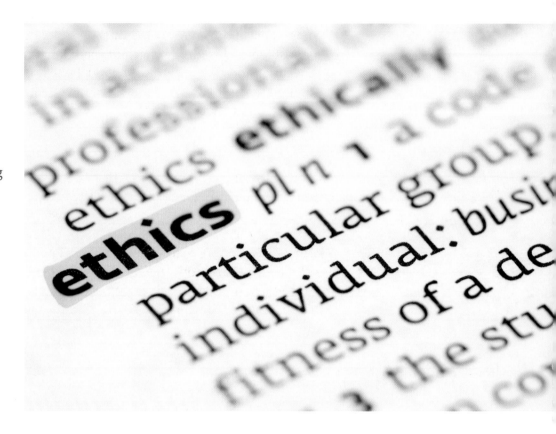

LEARNING OBJECTIVES

After reading this chapter, the student should be able to:

2.1 Compare and contrast law and ethics as they interface within the practice of dental hygiene.

2.2 Explain how the practice of dental hygiene is defined through statutory law and how a thorough understanding of the law is necessary.

2.3 Distinguish between criminal and civil law as they pertain to the practice of dental hygiene and strategies that assist in risk management.

2.4 Analyze how the ethical principal and core value of autonomy factors into both patient and provider autonomy.

2.5 Identify ways in which informed consent comes into play when discussing the issue of autonomy in health care.

2.6 Explore how dental hygiene professional organizations around the world address the issue of beneficence in their ethical codes and values, and discuss common themes.

2.7 Provide a rationale for how current access to health-care issues and beneficence interface, and develop strategies for addressing these issues.

2.8 Debate how nonmaleficence can lead to conflict when trying to balance good against harm for the same patient.

2.9 Explore the issue of justice through the eyes of legislators and policy makers who must grapple with issues of allocation of limited resources.

2.10 Define what is meant by a fiduciary relationship between patient and provider, and, in the context of the ethical principle and core value of veracity, discuss the idea of shared decision-making.

2.11 Evaluate the impact of the Health Insurance Portability and Accountability Act (HIPAA) on the ethical principle and core value of confidentiality.

2.12 Assess the factors that combine to create trust—for example, reciprocity, moral obligation, and trustworthiness—in the context of the practice of dentistry and dental hygiene, and compare with other health professions.

2.13 Use an ethical decision-making model when presented with an ethical dilemma to assist with critically thinking and problem-solving through an appropriate course of action.

KEY CONCEPTS

- As licensed health-care providers, the public places trust that the dental hygienist will practice legally and ethically.
- To practice legally and ethically, the dental hygienist must have a full understanding of ethical principles and core values and a full understanding of the law that will serve to guide decision-making.
- Use of an ethical decision-making model that incorporates professional codes of ethics, standards of care, and the law is key to critically thinking and problem-solving when faced with an ethical dilemma.

RELEVANCE TO CLINICAL PRACTICE

Martin Luther King said, "Intelligence is not enough . . . intelligence plus character—that is the true goal of education." Why discuss legal and ethical considerations in a dental hygiene textbook? In addition to developing clinical expertise, it is critical that dental hygiene students understand what it means legally to be a licensed practitioner and how ethics factor into the life and work of a health-care professional.

As in any health-care profession, legal and ethical issues arise in dentistry and dental hygiene. This chapter is devoted to introductory legal and ethical principles and their application to clinical practice. The **ethical decision-making** model is presented as a way to resolve ethical dilemmas. The American, Canadian, and International Dental Hygiene Code of Ethics are all presented.

The Basics

1. All of the following are functions of state dental boards *except* for one. Which one is the *exception?*
   A. Amendment of statutory law
   B. Requiring continuing education for licensees
   C. Determination of qualifications for applicants for a license to practice
   D. Enforcement of dental law to ensure the protection of the public

2. Fill in the blanks as to how a bill becomes a law in the United States.

| Both houses do not accept the bill. | |

| | Governor signs the bill into law. |

| Governor vetoes the bill. | |

3. Insert the correct term for each definition, which can be located in the American Dental Hygienists' Association (ADHA) code of ethics available at https://www.adha.org/resources-docs/7611_Bylaws_and_Code_of_Ethics.pdf.

   A. _____ requires the consideration of values and perspectives of others before making decisions or taking actions.

   B. _____ if an individual judges an action to be right or wrong, other people would make the same judgment considering the same action in the same situation.

4. Compare the two types of law by identifying the missing information.

	Criminal Law	Civil Law
Violation against:	_____	_____
Example of a dental hygiene violation:	_____	_____
Consequences:	_____	_____

5. List three areas addressed by dental hygiene statutory law.

   1) _____

   2) _____

   3) _____

6. After reviewing your patient's assessments with him, you discuss a treatment plan that will address his evident periodontal disease condition. Your patient insists that he does not have "gum disease" and demands that he be given a "regular cleaning." How does the patient's right to autonomy influence this situation? Do you as the dental hygienist have a right to autonomy?

_____

_____

_____

_____

_____

_____

_____

7. With regard to the seven principles of the privacy rule, describe these terms.

Rule	Meaning
Access	_____
Notice	_____
Onward transfer	_____

8. List the elements that should be included in your regular documentation practices.

_____

_____

_____

_____

_____

_____

_____

Learning Activities

1. Discuss why state lawmakers designate lawmaking power to agencies such as a state dental board.

_____

_____

_____

2. Identify a statement in the modern Hippocratic Oath and discuss how it relates to the practice of dental hygiene.

_____

_____

_____

_____

3. Relate societal trust to your interactions with a patient.

_____

_____

_____

_____

4. Create and present a scenario in which it would be appropriate for a dental hygienist to disclose protected health information (PHI).

_____

_____

_____

_____

Board Style Review Questions

1. Match the ethical principles and core values with the appropriate corresponding term.

__F__ Autonomy   A. nondisclosure

__B__ Beneficence   B. doing good

__A__ Confidentiality   C. do no harm

__D__ Justice   D. fairness

__C__ Nonmaleficence   E. honesty

__E__ Veracity   F. self-determination

2. All of the statements represent the term beneficence *except* for one. Which one is the *exception*?
   A. The dental hygienist should prevent harm to the patient.
   B. The dental hygienist should remove potential harm toward a patient.
   C. The dental hygienist should not cause harm to a patient.
   D. The dental hygienist should do good.

3. Dental practice acts and licensure are regulated by:
   A. Federal legislative law
   B. Judicial law
   C. Statutory law
   D. State legislative law
      1) A and B
      2) A and C
      3) B and D
      4) C and D

4. Which option best represents the concept of informed consent?
   A. Consulting the patient only when necessary
   B. Shared decision-making
   C. Paternalistic
   D. Decision-making is the responsibility of the practitioner
   E. None of the above

5. Professional liability insurance for a dental hygienist is not necessary as the hygienist is already covered under his/her dentist employer's liability insurance.
   A. The statement and the reason are both correct.
   B. The statement is correct, but the reason is incorrect.
   C. The statement and the reason are both incorrect.
   D. The statement is incorrect, but the reason is correct.

6. Choose the term that denotes a relationship between persons in which one person acts for another in a position of trust.
   A. Trust
   B. Justice
   C. Veracity
   D. Fiduciary

7. Under HIPAA, the individual has the right to request restrictions on the use or disclosure of their PHI. However, authorization from the individual is not required for the use and disclosure of PHI for the purpose of payment.
   A. Both statements are true.
   B. The first statement is true; the second is false.
   C. Both statements are false.
   D. The first statement is false; the second is true.

8. State dental practice acts are regulated under:
   1) Executive law
   2) Judicial law
   3) Legislative law
   4) Statutory law
      A. 1, 2, and 3
      B. 1 and 4
      C. 3 and 4
      D. All of the answers are correct

9. Order the steps in the decision-making model.

   _____ Apply the ethical principles to the options.

   _____ Determine whether the problem is in conflict with ethical principles.

   _____ Choose the best option, then implement.

   _____ Evaluate.

   _____ Gather credible resources and facts.

   _____ List options/alternatives.

10. The final HIPAA security rule applies to all PHI at covered entities. Hard drives, memory cards, Internet, and private networks are electronic devices covered under HIPAA.
    A. Both statements are correct
    B. The first statement is correct; the second is incorrect.
    C. Both statements are incorrect.
    D. The first statement is incorrect; the second statement is correct.

Resources

http://www.adha.org/governmental_affairs/practice_issues.htm.

Chapter 3 | Communication Skills

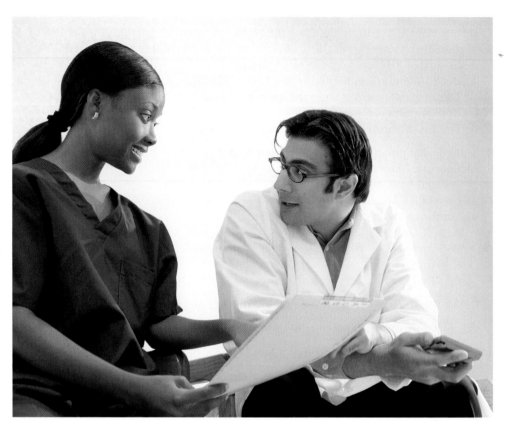

LEARNING OBJECTIVES

After reading this chapter, the student should be able to:

3.1 Discuss strategies for impactful communication throughout the dental hygiene process of care.

3.2 Outline ideal proxemics for optimal patient communication.

3.3 Describe various communication strategies for eliciting comprehensive information from a patient.

3.4 Detail the principles of motivational interviewing and how to apply them to clinical care.

3.5 Give examples of language strategies to create value for the dental hygiene process of care.

3.6 Discuss cultural differences and how they might apply to the dental hygiene process of care.

KEY CONCEPTS

• Communication skills are highly individualized from person to person.

• Some of the best communicators are first and foremost good listeners.

• Reflective listening is a critical skill that allows the dental hygienist to gather important information related to the individual patient.

- In addition to oral communication skills, current technology trends and generational preferences have spawned a new era of communication that uses platforms such as e-mail communication, text messaging, and social media websites.
- Communication proxemics is essential skills used during the dental hygiene appointment.
- Dental hygienists can set patients up for success while creating value for the dental hygiene appointment through compelling word choices.
- Motivational interviewing is a new strategy for enhancing the relationships between clinician and patient to better achieve adherence with treatment plans and long-term oral care protocols.
- With the increasingly diverse landscape of culture across the United States, cultural competency awareness is necessary for all dental hygiene professionals.

RELEVANCE TO CLINICAL PRACTICE

Communication is the cornerstone of almost every aspect of the dental hygienist's career. Productive, healthy communication occurs between the dental staff and the dentist, between individual staff members, between clinicians and patients, and between clinicians and patient caregivers (i.e., parents of minors, spouses, home health aides, etc.). For behavior change to occur, patients must feel a connection with the dental professional. Connections are made through strategic, purposeful listening and dialogue tactics that allow for clinicians to establish common ground with patients, essentially humanizing themselves to break through the sterile relationship of health-care provider and patient.

The Basics

1. Choose one of the following clinical suggestion that would provide the most success in communicating if your patient is from a high power/distance culture.
   A. Involve as many people as possible in decision-making.
   B. Ask the dentist to participate in clinical recommendations.
   C. Do not ask for too much personal information.
   D. Encourage dialogue and expression of the patient's own ideas.

2. Choose one of the following clinical suggestions that would provide the most success in communicating if your patient is from a culture with a low uncertainty/avoidance index.
   A. Introduce change slowly.
   B. Treat men and women equally.
   C. Express your emotions through hand gestures and voice inflection.
   D. Express curiosity when you discover differences.

3. Oral communication is influenced by:

1) _____

2) _____

3) _____

4) _____

5) _____

6) _____

4. All of the following terms influence communication. Identify the terms that influence nonverbal communication.

1) Tone   4) Speed

2) Hand gestures   5) Clarity

3) Body movements   6) Facial expressions

5. The listener relies on the following cues to interpret what the speaker has said.

1) 55% are determined by: _____

2) 38% are determined by: _____

3) 7% are determined by: _____

6. Explain the importance of understanding "who" your patient is before providing oral hygiene instruction.

_____

_____

_____

_____

7. The effectiveness of written communication depends on the preferences of the speaker. The effectiveness also depends on the appropriateness of the vocabulary used, grammar, and conciseness.
   A. Both statements are true.
   B. The first statement is true; the second is false.
   C. Both statements are false.
   D. The first statement is false; the second statement is true.

8. List the three components that convey meaning in face-to-face verbal communication.

1) _____

2) _____

3) _____

Learning Activities

1. Create a scenario that communicates value to the patient when it comes to rescheduling a recare/recall appointment.

_____

_____

_____

_____

2. Practice motivational interviewing with a student partner.

3. Practice improving your verbal and nonverbal cues with a student partner.

4. Give examples of how to use nonverbal communication through pictorial representation during oral hygiene instruction.

_____

_____

_____

Board Style Review Questions

1. Match the five key dimensions of culture with the corresponding definition.

_____ Power/distance	A. strength of the ties people have to others within the community
_____ Individualism	B. degree of anxiety society members feel in unknown situations
_____ Masculinity	C. how much society values long-standing traditions and values
_____ Uncertainty/Avoidance Index	D. how much society values traditional male and female roles
_____ Long-term Orientation	E. degree of inequality that exists and is accepted

2. Which of the following measurements represents the close proximity phase for personal distance?
   A. Less than 6 inches
   B. 1.5 to 2.5 feet
   C. 4 to 7 feet
   D. 12 to 25 feet

3. Which of the following measurements represents the close proximity phase for social distance?
   A. Less than 6 inches
   B. 1.5 to 2.5 feet
   C. 4 to 7 feet
   D. 12 to 25 feet

4. During dental hygiene treatment, what distance zone represents patient-operator proximity?
   A. Intimate
   B. Personal
   C. Social
   D. Public
       1) A and B
       2) A and C
       3) B and C
       4) C and D

5. All of the following *except* one are explanations as to why it might appear that your patient has not "listened" to your recommendations from the last dental hygiene appointment. Which one is the *exception?*
   A. The message you presented was too lengthy and/or complex.
   B. The message used culturally insensitive language.
   C. The message was audible.
   D. The message contained grammatical errors.

6. Patients may feel apprehensive during a dental hygiene appointment and withhold information because:
   A. They may not believe the information is pertinent to the appointment.
   B. They may be embarrassed about sharing private information.
   C. They may not have been asked these questions at a previous appointment so they do not think it is necessary to answer them now.
   D. All of these could be reasons for patients to withhold information.

7. A patient says, "I want to brush better, but I am always in a hurry to get to work." This is an example of:
   A. Ambivalence
   B. Autonomy
   C. Motivational interviewing
   D. Reflective listening

8. Reflective listening is:
   A. A one-way feedback loop of communication between the patient and clinician and vice versa.
   B. A collaborative, person-centered form of guiding to elicit and strengthen motivation to change.
   C. Imparting or exchanging thoughts, opinions, or information.
   D. A two-way feedback loop of communication.

9. Which option is not one of the three pillars of motivational interviewing?
   A. Autonomy
   B. Collaboration
   C. Dependence
   D. Evocation

10. Traditional oral health education consists of giving advice to patients and persuading patients to adopt these approaches. Motivational interviewing uses more of a collaborative approach where the dental hygienist helps to guide and motivate the patient for change.
    A. Both statements are correct.
    B. The first statement is correct; the second is incorrect.
    C. Both statements are incorrect.
    D. The first statement is incorrect; the second statement is correct.

Active Learning

Theresa is a dental hygienist practicing at Winding Oaks Dental Office. She checks her computer monitor to confirm the time of her next patient. The schedule shows that her next patient, Mr. Donald, has cancelled his appointment. Theresa finishes preparing her operatory for the afternoon and checks to see if she can assist any of the other clinicians. She then reports to the clinic manager to let her know that her patient has cancelled and she will be working on organizing the inventory downstairs. Fifteen minutes later the front office administration is frantically looking for Theresa because Mr. Donald is irritated that he has been waiting so long to be seen. Theresa explains to the office administrator that her schedule showed that he had cancelled the appointment. Theresa rushes out to the reception area to escort Mr. Donald back to the operatory. She waves him in and apologizes for keeping him waiting. Theresa is reviewing Mr. Donald's health history while she is putting on her loupes and mask. Theresa discusses updating his radiographs per the treatment plan. Theresa asks if he agrees to the radiographs and Mr. Donald nods his head, yes. While Theresa is exposing the radiographs, she asks Mr. Donald if he has been using the Proxabrush® she provided at his last visit. Mr. Donald states "no." Use this case scenario to answer these questions.

1. What concerns, if any, are there with Theresa donning her personal protective equipment while reviewing the medical history?
   A. There are no concerns as Theresa is multitasking.
   B. The patient is not in the ideal position to assess Theresa's body language.
   C. The clinician is in the patient's personal distance.
   D. Theresa's communication with the patient is not efficient.

2. Nonverbal communication was used when:
    1) Theresa discussed the cancellation with the clinic manager.
    2) Theresa apologized to Mr. Donald.
    3) Theresa waved Mr. Donald back toward the operatory.
    4) Mr. Donald nodded his head.
       A. 1 and 2
       B. 2 and 3
       C. 3 and 4
       D. 3

3. Mr. Donald states "no" when Theresa asks him if he is using the Proxabrush®. This is an example of which type of communication?
    A. Closed-ended question
    B. Motivational interviewing
    C. Open-ended dialogue
    D. One-way communication loop

4. Team-Based Learning: In a small group, discuss how the communication between dental team members could be improved.

_____

_____

_____

_____

_____

_____

_____

_____

_____

_____

_____

_____

_____

_____

_____

_____

_____

_____

_____

_____

_____

_____

_____

_____

_____

_____

_____

_____

Rubrics/Process Evaluations

Process Evaluation Template		
Communication Assessment		
Evaluation Criteria	**Criteria Met? (Y/N)**	**Comments**
Student uses appropriate nonverbal cues when greeting patient (smiles, extends hand, walks with confidence).		
Student maintains ideal positioning during multitasking to allow patient to assess clinician's body language.		
Student uses nonverbal communication through pictorial representation during patient education.		
Student uses a personal or social distance when communicating an important message to the patient.		
Messages between the student and patient are generally of reasonable length, complexity, audible, and grammatically correct.		
Culturally sensitive language was implemented and consideration was given to the five key dimensions of culture.		
Open-ended questions were used as opposed to close-ended questions.		
Motivational interviewing was incorporated.		
Reflective listening was utilized.		
Student uses Standard Precautions.		

Part II

The Dental Hygienist's Role in the Delivery of Health Care

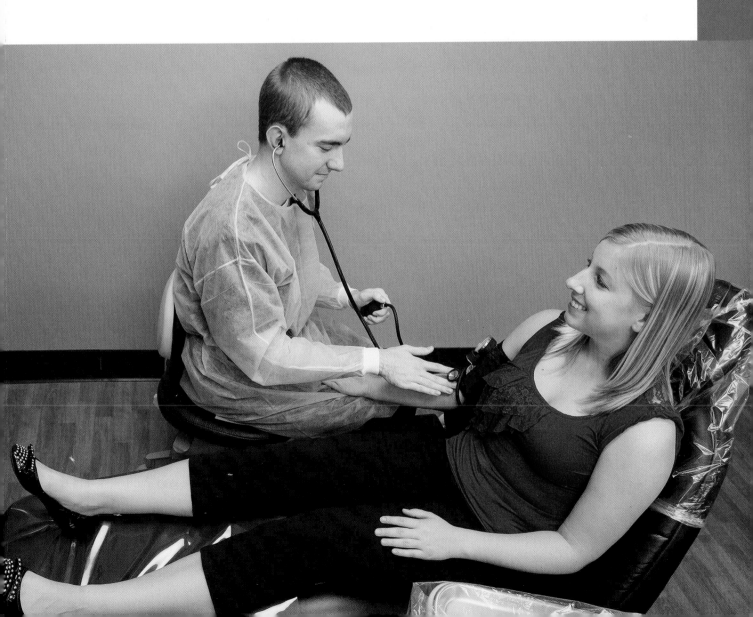

Chapter 4 | Health Education and Promotion

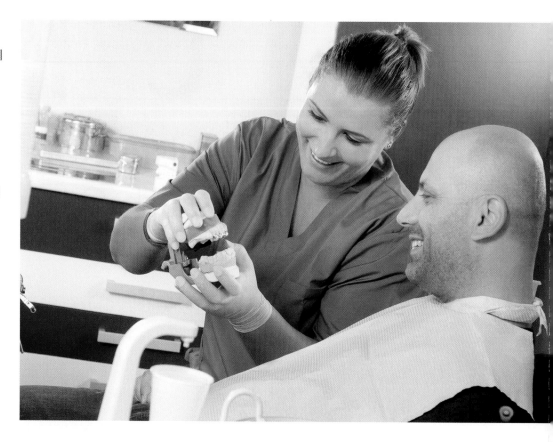

LEARNING OBJECTIVES

After reading this chapter, the student should be able to:

4.1 Discuss disparities in oral health care.

4.2 Distinguish between health and wellness.

4.3 Explain similarities and differences between education for prevention and education for promotion.

4.4 Compare and contrast health-promotion strategies.

4.5 Assess, plan, implement, and evaluate oral health behavior change using health-promotion strategies.

4.6 Differentiate health-promotion strategies for the child, adolescent, and adult.

4.7 Implement tobacco cessation strategies as appropriate.

KEY CONCEPTS

• Dental hygienists contribute to their patients' health and wellness by providing holistic care.

• Dental hygienists help patients achieve optimal health and wellness through health promotion and education.

• In the United States, the cost of health care and lack of health insurance coverage limits accessibility to health care for a large number of people.

The Affordable Care Act makes dental insurance coverage available to all children and does not require parents to enroll children to gain coverage. For adults, some health plans will include dental coverage and some will not.

- Health education and health-promotion models include Maslow's hierarchy of needs, the learning ladder, the health belief model, and the transtheoretical model. To be effective, dental hygienists must be comfortable with a variety of models and utilize the model most appropriate for individual patients and their needs.
- Health education and promotion can be applied to every step of the dental hygiene process of care.
- Prevention and health-promotion models can be adapted to any age group. When providing health education, it is important to look at the motivating factors that are relevant to that age and to use age-appropriate language.
- Behavior modification models are effective for encouraging patients to adopt positive health behaviors and to eliminate negative health behaviors such as smoking. Patients must make the decision and commit to change to be successful.

RELEVANCE TO CLINICAL PRACTICE

Many systemic and oral diseases in the United States could be prevented with lifestyle changes. Modifying lifestyle by daily exercise, improving dietary habits, and decreasing tobacco use would help prevent many of the diseases that cause premature death and would decrease the prevalence of oral diseases.[1] As preventive oral health professionals, dental hygienists identify their patients' health risks and provide health education, motivation, and health promotion. The dental hygiene appointment offers an opportunity to discuss the relationship among the patient's oral conditions, what was reported on the medical history, and other information provided. As respected professionals in the community, dental hygienists also provide health-promotion services at schools, health fairs, or other community events.

The Basics

1. Choose the best statement to define Motivational Interviewing (MI).
   A. A health-promotion technique that has shown a positive relationship to behavior change.
   B. An individual's readiness to change for improved health.
   C. A behavioral model focusing on the individual's intent.
   D. Identifying a patient's level of knowledge.

2. What is the key to behavior change?
   A. Knowledge
   B. Awareness
   C. Motivation
   D. Education

3. List and define the six stages of the transtheoretical model.

1) _____

_____

_____

2) _____

_____

_____

3) _____

_____

_____

4) _____

_____

_____

5) _____

_____

_____

6) _____

_____

_____

4. Which term identifies a person who does not believe that they can make a change but would be more willing to try if a reward is offered?
A. Internal locus of control
B. External locus of control
C. Theory of Reasoned Action
D. Self-efficacy

5. Select the true statement related to smoking cessation for adolescents.
A. Cigarette smoking increased among middle school and high school youth between 2000 and 2011.
B. Youth are more likely to smoke if they have a strong racial identity.
C. The use of electronic cigarettes and hookah pipes has increased.
D. Youth are less likely to smoke if they lack parental support.

6. Prevention and health-promotion models will be effective with the elderly when:
A. Education is generalized to the elderly population.
B. The dental hygienist focuses only on oral health.
C. The emphasis is placed on social consequences.
D. The education is relevant and individualized.

7. The dental hygienist should adapt prevention and health-promotion models to the adolescent's stage of development. It is suggested that health promotion would be more effective if the emphasis were placed on health consequences rather than social consequences.
A. Both statements are true.
B. The first statement is true; the second is false.
C. Both statements are false.
D. The first statement is false; the second statement is true.

8. Label the components of the acronym S.T.A.R.T. as related to the tobacco cessation process.

S = _____

T = _____

A = _____

R = _____

T = _____

Learning Activities

1. Name two issues that could affect the quality of health care in the United States.

_____

_____

_____

_____

_____

_____

2. Discuss some of the circumstances that contribute to disparities in access to health care.

_____

_____

_____

_____

_____

_____

3. Analyze the objectives outlined in Healthy People 2020. Describe the dental hygienist's role in improving health as related to these objectives.

_____

_____

_____

_____

_____

_____

Board Style Review Questions

1. Identify one of the following that is not a part of the "5 A's" of The American Dental Hygienists Association's National Smoking Cessation Initiative.
   A. Ask
   B. Advise
   C. Assess
   D. Alter

2. A state of complete physical, mental, and social well-being and not merely the absence of disease is:
   A. Wellness
   B. Health
   C. Holistic care
   D. Health promotion

3. All of the following are constructs of the Health Belief Model *except* for one. Which one is the *exception?*
   A. The individual's beliefs about the probability of developing a condition.
   B. The person is not thinking about change.
   C. The individual's beliefs about how serious a condition is if it does develop.
   D. Exposure to information that motivates the individual to act.

4. The belief in one's capabilities to organize and execute the courses of action required to manage prospective situations is:
   A. Social cognitive theory
   B. Self-efficacy
   C. Locus of control
   D. Health belief

5. An individual's beliefs about what factors determine his or her rewards or outcomes in life is referred to as:
   A. Social cognitive theory
   B. Self-efficacy
   C. Locus of control
   D. Health belief

6. Which health-promotion model was originally used for smoking cessation but can also be used for implementing positive behavior, such as flossing?
   A. Transtheoretical/stages of change model
   B. Learning ladder
   C. Maslow's hierarchy of needs
   D. Health belief model

7. The process in which a patient is unaware of a condition, becomes aware of the condition, and then decides how this new information applies to him/her is part of the:
   A. Transtheoretical/stages of change model
   B. Learning ladder
   C. Maslow's hierarchy of needs
   D. Health belief model

8. Which of the following describes Maslow's hierarchy of needs?
   A. A model to evaluate the stage where an individual is on a continuum related to making a behavioral change.
   B. An individual characteristic that may influence all of the models for behavior change.
   C. A theory focusing on the individual's intent.
   D. Influential for increasing understanding of readiness to change behavior.

9. The process of enabling people to increase control over their health is called:
   A. Health education
   B. Health promotion
   C. Holistic care
   D. Paternalism

10. Traditional oral health education consists of giving advice to patients and persuading the patient to adopt these approaches. Motivational interviewing uses more of a collaborative approach where the dental hygienist helps to guide and motivate the patient for change.
    A. Both statements are correct.
    B. The first statement is correct; the second is incorrect.
    C. Both statements are incorrect.
    D. The first statement is incorrect; the second statement is correct.

REFERENCES

1. Danaei G, Ding EL, Mozffarian D, Taylor B, Rehm J, Murray CJ, Ezzati M. The preventable causes of death in the United States: comparative risk assessment of dietary, lifestyle and metabolic risk factors. *PLoS Med.* 2009;6(4):e10000058.

Rubrics/Process Evaluations

Process Evaluation Template		
Health Education and Promotion		
Evaluation Criteria	**Criteria Met? (Y/N)**	**Comments**
Assessment: Student observes the patient's gait, skin color, etc., to gather information.		
Dental Hygiene Diagnosis: Student uses assessments to determine issues that need attention through education and health promotion.		
Planning: Student collaborates with patient to discuss health issues that require behavior change. (Patient decides what to do.)		
Implementation: Student educates the patient, involves the patient in setting goals.		
Evaluation: Student uses measurable criteria to evaluate the patient's progress toward achieving goals, and communicates outcomes to patient and other providers. Determines next step and revision of goals as needed.		
Documentation: Document each step of the dental hygiene process of care including all information.		

Chapter 5 | Immunology and the Oral Systemic Link

KEY TERMS

active immunity

adaptive or acquired
    immune response

antigen–antibody
    complex

bacteremia

complement cascade

complement system

C-reactive protein (CRP)

cytokine

differential gene
    expression

glucometer

innate immune response

innate susceptibility

interleukin

lipoxin

matrix metalloproteinase
    (MMP)

meta-analyses

nosocomial pneumonia

passive immunity

periodontal medicine

phagocytes

polymorphonuclear
    neutrophil (PNM)

resolvins

risk factor

vaccination

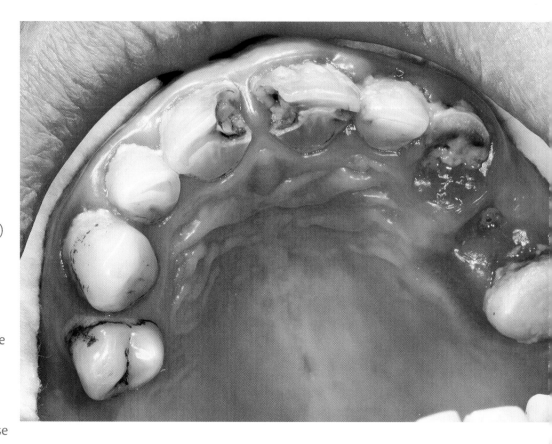

LEARNING OBJECTIVES

After reading this chapter, the student should be able to:

5.1 Describe the immune system and how it works.

5.2 Illustrate new concepts in the etiology and pathogenesis of periodontal diseases.

5.3 Distinguish the risk factors for periodontal disease.

5.4 Appraise the research regarding the connection between oral and systemic disease.

5.5 Examine the steps in co-management of periodontal and related systemic disease.

5.6 Enhance understanding of bacteremia associated with periodontal diseases.

5.7 Explain the link between oral and systemic disease to the patient.

KEY CONCEPTS

- Considerable epidemiological evidence to support the concept that poor oral health, especially the extent and severity of periodontal disease, may put patients at a significant risk for a variety of systemic conditions.
- There is increasing evidence that reducing the inflammatory component of the disease in periodontal tissue disease has potential systemic effects.

• Reducing the inflammatory burden in the periodontal tissues has been shown to improve the progression of periodontal diseases, improve hyperglycemic control in diabetics, and improve surrogate markers that may be of benefit in patients suffering from coronary heart disease

RELEVANCE TO CLINICAL PRACTICE

Oral diseases and infections are a major public health problem worldwide, in spite of advances in understanding, prevention, and treatment of gingivitis and chronic periodontitis. They are still among the most prevalent microbial diseases of mankind.[1] As demographics change, and the number of people retaining their natural teeth increases, there is also an increased risk for periodontal disease (PD). The mouth is a significant contributor to the total burden of infection and inflammation, and consequently, to overall health and well-being. This chapter will review the role the immune system plays in periodontal infection, the link between oral health and systemic health, and the theories that support this connection.

The term **periodontal medicine** refers to the role of systemic factors on PD, and the association of PD with chronic diseases of aging such as diabetes and cardiovascular disease (CVD).[2] The relationship between oral health and general health has been increasingly recognized over recent years, and a number of epidemiological studies have now linked poor oral health with CVD, poor glycemic control in diabetics, respiratory diseases, rheumatoid arthritis, and osteoporosis. Systemic conditions may increase the susceptibility to periodontal disease, and conversely, periodontal infections may serve as risk factors for systemic illness. A **risk factor** is any attribute, characteristic, or exposure of an individual that increases the likelihood of developing a disease or injury. Some examples of the more important risk factors are underweight, unsafe sex, high blood pressure, tobacco and alcohol consumption, and unsafe water, sanitation, and hygiene.[3] The relationship between oral and general health is a significant issue, and it should lead to more aggressive prevention and management of PD, and co-management of patients with other health care professionals

The Basics
1. Which immune defense response provides immediate protection against invading pathogens?
    A. Acquired immune response
    B. Adaptive immune response
    C. Artificially acquired response
    D. Innate immune response

2. Which immune defense response confers specificity and long-lasting protection?
   A. Acquired immune response
   B. Artificially acquired response
   C. Innate immune response
   D. Natural immune response

3. Active immunity usually lasts a few months. Passive immunity lasts much longer, sometimes lifelong.
   A. Both statements are correct.
   B. The first statement is correct; the second statement is incorrect.
   C. Both statements are incorrect.
   D. The first statement is incorrect; the second statement is correct.

4. All are characteristics of the complement cascade system *except* for one. Which one is the *exception?*
   A. Clears pathogens from an organism
   B. Rids the body of antigen-antibody complexes
   C. Triggered when the first complement molecule encounters an antibody bound to an antigen
   D. Assists the antibodies in maintaining bacteria

5. Chemical messengers of the immune system are:
   A. Antigens
   B. Cytokines
   C. Matrix metalloproteinases
   D. Resolvins

6. Define periodontal medicine.

   _____

   _____

   _____

   _____

7. All blood cells come from:
   A. Bone marrow
   B. Fibroblasts
   C. Lipoxins
   D. Matrix metalloproteinases

8. A number of studies have shown that the periodontitis lesion involves predominantly:
   A. Plasma cells
   B. T cells
   C. B cells

9. List the potential outcomes of reducing the inflammatory burden in the periodontal tissues.

   1) _____

   _____

   _____

   2) _____

   _____

   _____

   3) _____

   _____

   _____

Learning Activities

1. Discuss the risk factors for periodontal disease.

_____

_____

_____

_____

_____

_____

_____

_____

_____

_____

_____

_____

2. Locate a research article related to the connection between oral and systemic disease. Use evidence-based decision-making to evaluate the article.

   Article title and author:

_____

   Evaluation:

_____

_____

_____

_____

3. Role-play with a student partner. Explain the link between oral and systemic diseases to a patient. Notes:

_____

_____

_____

Board Style Review Questions

1. Match the lymphoid organ with the appropriate descriptor.

   _____ adenoids   A. Two oval masses in the back of the throat

   _____ appendix   B. Two lobes in front of the trachea

   _____ bone marrow   C. Two glands located at the back of the nasal passage

   _____ lymph nodes   D. Fist-sized organ located in the abdominal cavity

   _____ spleen   E. Small organs that connect via lymphatic vessels

   _____ thymus   F. Small tube that is connected to the large intestines

   _____ tonsils   G. Soft, fatty tissue found in bone cavities

2. Which of the following are responsible for increased collagen breakdown?
   A. Polymorphonuclear neutrophils
   B. Tumor necrosis factor alpha
   C. Matrix metalloproteinases

3. Which of the following fatty acids help in the resolution of inflammation?
   1) Cytokines
   2) Lipoxins
   3) Resolvins
   4) Neutrophils
      A. 1 and 2
      B. 1 and 3
      C. 2 and 3
      D. 3 and 4

4. What determines the ultimate outcome of the periodontal disease process?
   A. Innate susceptibility of the host
   B. Adaptive immunity of the host
   C. Disease modifiers
   D. Disease resolution

5. A C-reactive protein test is an additional way to assess:
   A. Diabetes risk
   B. Cardiovascular disease risk
   C. Innate susceptibility
   D. Adaptive immunity

6. The C-reactive protein (CRP) risk group that represents an average risk is:
   A. 0.1 mg/L
   B. 0.9 mg/L
   C. 2.0 mg/L
   D. 3.0 mg/L

7. Which is *not* a characteristic of complement proteins?
   A. Assist antibodies in destroying bacteria
   B. Cause blood vessels to constrict
   C. Cause redness and swelling during an inflammatory response
   D. Circulate in the blood

8. All of the following are cytokines *except* for one. Which one is the *exception?*
   A. Growth factors
   B. Interleukins
   C. Interferons
   D. B cells

9. The immune defense acquired through transfer of antibodies is referred to as:
   A. Active immunity
   B. Innate immunity
   C. Passive immunity
   D. Transient immunity

10. The innate/adaptive immune cells originate in:
    A. Bone marrow
    B. Growth factors
    C. Lymph nodes
    D. White blood cells

REFERENCES

1. Seymour GJ, Ford PJ, Cullinan MP, Leishman S, West MJ, Yamazaki K. Infection or inflammation: the link between periodontal and cardiovascular diseases. *Future Cardiol.* 2009;5(1):5-9.
2. Genco RJ, Williams RC. *Periodontal Disease and Overall Health: A Clinician's Guide.* Yardley, PA: Professional Audience Communications, Inc.; 2010:48.
3. World Health Organization. Risk factors. Available from: http://www.who.int/topics/risk_factors/en. Accessed May 27, 2014.

Chapter 6 | Evidence-Based Care

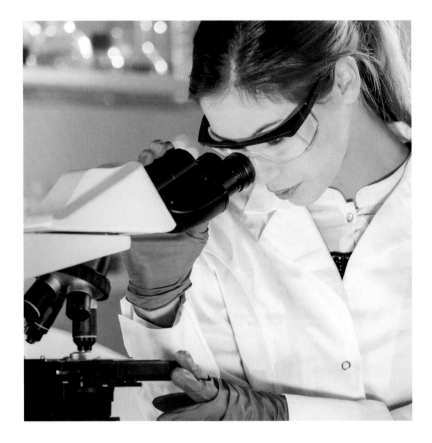

LEARNING OBJECTIVES

After reading this chapter, the student should be able to:

6.1 Define *evidence-based care*.

6.2 Discuss the principles of evidence-based care.

6.3 Describe the methods of the evidence-based process.

6.4 Explain the importance and hierarchy of the evidence-based process.

6.5 Apply evidence-based decision-making to patient care.

6.6 Perform a basic search for and evaluation of scientific literature.

6.7 Write a basic scientific paper.

KEY CONCEPTS

• Evidence-based care (EBC) is based on three tenets and is only considered
  to be actively in use when *all* three tenets have been incorporated into the
  process of care.

• The three tenets are: (a) the best available scientific evidence; (b) a
  clinician's skill, judgment, and experience; and (c) consideration for the
  patient's needs, preferences, values, and beliefs. Evidence alone does not
  replace sound clinical judgment. However, the hierarchical levels of quality
  and valid evidence aid in the clinical decision-making process. The dental
  hygiene process of care is based on a critical thinking model and the focus
  is on provision of patient-centered, comprehensive care.

- As dental hygienists perform the roles of clinician, educator, researcher, manager, and advocate to prevent oral disease and promote overall health, it is imperative that they remain scientifically up-to-date to answer the needs of their patients.

RELEVANCE TO CLINICAL PRACTICE

Dental hygienists are required to make informed decisions about patient care. Careful examination of scientific research allows clinicians, together with their patients, to make **best practice** decisions about that care. **Evidence-based care (EBC)** is a patient-centered approach to care, merging the best available research with clinical expertise and patient preferences.[1–6] It serves as a blueprint for health professionals as they make patient care decisions to ensure the best health outcomes. **Evidence-based decision-making** requires critical thinking and research skills.[1–7] Dental hygienists must be proficient at locating, interpreting, and appropriately applying scientific evidence to support their patient care decision-making.

Patients look to oral health professionals not only for clinical care but for answers to questions and to verify information obtained via the Internet or other sources. Due to the vast number of research articles published annually, it can be difficult for oral health professionals to keep abreast of current research findings.[8] The amount of new research may cause variations in dental hygiene practice. Variations can occur from the lack of integration of new knowledge into practice, reliance on traditional passive methods of continuing education and the absence of active searches for **empirical evidence**, incorrect interpretation or evaluation of new information, and poor or lack of scientific evidence required to answer specific clinical questions.[9–11] The same technological advancements have changed the way oral health-care professionals seek and gather information. Knowing how to efficiently and effectively conduct searches for scientific evidence and critically appraising it will yield valid information for answering clinical and patient questions, and providing the best care to patients.

Evidence-based dental hygiene care requires the skills of efficient, systematic literature searches and application of the rules of evidence to critically evaluate the clinical literature. A **systematic search** is a strategized tactic for locating answers to clinical and other questions by mining scientific and biomedical databases.[7,9,12] A good clinical question starts the process.[3,12–16] It formally introduces the patient, who presents with a problem. Second, it promotes more questioning, which helps to formulate the principal question and pinpoints the issue. Finally, a good clinical question defines and refines the evidence search strategy. The purpose of a systematic literature search is to identify potentially relevant articles. Evaluating the evidence critically reveals the validity and the pertinence of a study.[7,16,17] Clinically relevant research that has been conducted using reliable methodology provides the best evidence.[7,16,17]

The Basics

1. All of the following are correct as related to statistical significance *except* for one. Which one is the *exception?*
   A. It is expressed as a *p* value.
   B. It refers to the level of significance.
   C. It is the only factor to consider for patient care decision-making.
   D. It is the level of probability that an association between two or more variables occurred by chance alone.

2. Which type of research question is best investigated with a randomized controlled trial?
   1) Dental hygiene diagnosis
   2) Dental hygiene prevention
   3) Dental hygiene prognosis
   4) Dental hygiene therapy
      A. 1 and 4
      B. 2 and 3
      C. 2 and 4
      D. 3 and 4

3. Primary research is considered clinical or basic research. Primary research includes literature reviews and meta-analyses.
   A. Both statements are true.
   B. The first statement is true; the second is false.
   C. Both statements are false.
   D. The first statement is false; the second is true.

4. Which type of study examines a large population and follows it over time?
   A. Case control
   B. Case series
   C. Cohort
   D. Randomized controlled trial

5. Choose the study that represents the highest level of evidence.
   A. Case control
   B. Case series
   C. Cohort
   D. Randomized controlled trial

6. Choose the statement that best defines reliability.
   A. Relevance and pertinence of the study in relation to the patient.
   B. The observed results occurred entirely by chance.
   C. The extent to which a study repeatedly and consistently produces the same outcome.
   D. The extent to which a study measures what it intends to measure.

7. List the six steps involved in the evidence-based process.

1) _____

_____

_____

2) _____

_____

_____

3) _____

_____

_____

4) _____

_____

_____

5) _____

_____

_____

6) _____

_____

_____

8. Identify the components of an abstract of a scientific paper.

1) _____

_____

_____

2) _____

_____

_____

3) _____

_____

_____

4) _____

_____

_____

5) _____

_____

_____

6) _____

_____

_____

Learning Activities

1. Explain the purpose of a literature review.

_____

_____

_____

_____

_____

_____

_____

_____

_____

_____

2. Describe the phases of the research writing process.

_____

_____

_____

_____

_____

_____

_____

_____

_____

_____

_____

3. Explain how the three tenets of evidence-based care should be incorporated into the process of care.

_____

_____

_____

_____

_____

_____

_____

_____

_____

_____

_____

Board Style Review Questions

1. The structure for the research strategy is provided by:
   A. A good clinical question
   B. A concise and exhaustive summary of the literature
   C. Merging the best available research
   D. Evaluating the evidence critically

2. Randomization is *not:*
   A. A study control method
   B. Researchers assign participants to an experimental or control group
   C. A haphazard assignment
   D. Performed using a carefully planned strategy

3. An open-label study can be described as a study in which:
   A. Both the participant and researcher are cognizant of the intervention.
   B. The participant is unaware of the intervention.
   C. Neither participant nor researcher is informed about the intervention.
   D. The researcher is aware of what the intervention will be.

4. A study that starts with an exposure and follows the patients forward to an outcome is a:
   A. Case control study
   B. Case series
   C. Prospective cohort study
   D. Retrospective cohort study

5. Studies in which participants are selected based on their disease and compared with people who do not have the disease are called:
   A. Randomized control studies
   B. Case control studies
   C. Case series
   D. Cohort

6. The commonly accepted *p* value is:
   A. ≤ 0.01
   B. ≤ 0.05
   C. ≤ 0.10
   D. ≤ 0.50

7. Choose the statement that best defines validity.
   A. Relevance and pertinence of the study in relation to the patient
   B. The observed results occurred entirely by chance
   C. Extent to which a study repeatedly and consistently produces the same outcome
   D. The extent to which a study measures what it intends to measure

8. Choose the best type of study for investigating a research question that involves a dental hygiene diagnosis.
   A. Case control
   B. Retrospective
   C. Randomized control trial
   D. Prospective

9. A strategy for locating answers to clinical and other questions by mining scientific and biomedical databases is called:
   A. Levels of evidence
   B. Evidence-based care
   C. Empirical evidence
   D. Systematic search

10. A study in which at least one group of participants receives an intervention while the other group receives a standard of care is referred to as a:
    A. Randomized control trial
    B. Cohort
    C. Case series
    D. Case control

REFERENCES

1. About EBD. Chicago: ADA Center for Evidence-Based Dentistry; 2013. Available from: http://ebd.ada.org/about.aspx. Accessed May 6, 2013.

2. EBD Educational Tutorials. Series on evidence-based dentistry. Chicago: ADA Center for Evidence-Based Dentistry; 2013. Available from: http://ebd.ada.org/VideoTutorials.aspx. Accessed May 6, 2013.

3. Guyatt G, Meade MO. How to use the medical literature—and this book—to improve your patient care. In: Guyatt G, Rennie D, Meade MO, Cook DJ, eds. *User's Guide to Medical Literature: A Manual for Evidence-Based Clinical Practice.* 2nd ed. Toronto, ON: McGraw-Hill; 2008:1-4.

4. Centre for Evidence-Based Medicine. Oxford, U.K.: University of Oxford; 2011. Available from: http://www.cebm.net/index.aspx?o=1914. Accessed September 30, 2013.

5. Ross T. Evidence-based practice. In: *A Survival Guide for Health Research Methods.* New York: McGraw-Hill; 2012:5-19.

6. What is evidence-based practice (EBP)? Durham, NC: Introduction to Evidence-Based Practice; 2013. Available from: http://guides.mclibrary.duke.edu/content.php?pid=431451&sid=3529499. Accessed September 30, 2013.

7. Selecting the resources. Durham, NC: Introduction to Evidence-Based Practice; 2013. Available from: http://guides.mclibrary.duke.edu/content.php?pid=431451&sid=3530457. Accessed September 30, 2013.

8. Bastian H, Glasziou P, Chlamers I. Seventy-five trials and eleven systematic reviews a day: how will we ever keep up? *PLoS Med.* 2010;7(9):1-6.

9. Faggion CM Jr. The development of evidence-based guidelines in dentistry. *J Dent Educ.* 2013;77(2):124-136.

10. Marshal TA, Straub-Morarend CL, Qian F, Finkelstein MW. Perceptions and practices of dental school faculty regarding evidence-based dentistry. *J Dent Educ.* 2013;77(2):146-151.

11. Palcanis KG, Geiger BF, O'Neal MR, Ivankova N, Retta RE, Kennedy LB, Carera KW. Preparing students to practice evidence-based dentistry: a mixed methods conceptual framework for curriculum enhancement. *J Dent Educ.* 2012;76(12):1600-1614.

12. Acquiring the evidence. Durham, NC: Introduction to Evidence-Based Practice; 2013. Available from: http://guides.mclibrary.duke.edu/content.php?pid=431451&sid=3530449. Accessed September 30, 2013.

13. Asking the well built clinical question. Durham, NC: Introduction to Evidence-Based Practice; 2013. Available from: http://guides.mclibrary.duke.edu/content.php?pid=431451&sid=3529524. Accessed September 30, 2013.

14. Type of question. Durham, NC: Introduction to Evidence-Based Practice; 2013. Available from: http://guides.mclibrary.duke.edu/content.php?pid=431451&sid=3530451. Accessed September 30, 2013.

15. Centre for Evidence-Based Medicine. Oxford, U.K.: University of Oxford; 2009. Available from: http://www.cebm.net/index.aspx?o=1036. Accessed September 30, 2013.

16. Type of study. Durham, NC: Introduction to Evidence-Based Practice; 2013. Available from: http://guides.mclibrary.duke.edu/content.php?pid=431451&sid=3530453. Accessed September 30, 2013.

17. Evaluating the validity of a therapy study. Durham, NC: Introduction to Evidence-Based Practice; 2013. Available from: http://guides.mclibrary.duke.edu/content.php?pid=431451&sid=3718368. Accessed September 30, 2013.

Part III

Infection Control

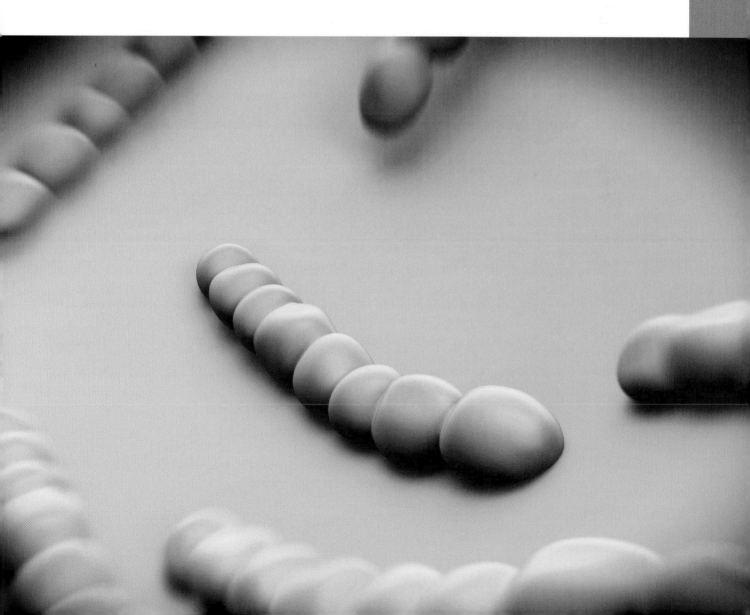

Chapter 7 | Exposure and Infection Control

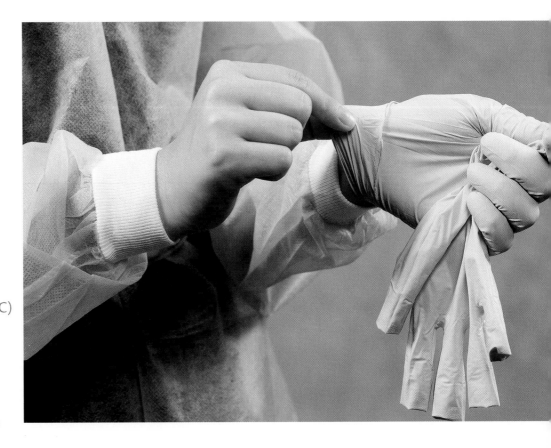

LEARNING OBJECTIVES

After reading this chapter, the student should be able to:

7.1 Discuss infectious diseases in terms of the infectious disease process and interventions to prevent disease transmission.

7.2 Outline initial intervention procedures of an occupational exposure, screening tests, and postexposure prophylaxis for HIV, hepatitis B, and hepatitis C.

7.3 Use critical thinking skills in the implementation of infection-control practices.

7.4 Explain the difference between nonregulated and regulated medical waste and infectious waste.

7.5 Integrate the environmentally responsible choices into infection-control practices.

KEY CONCEPTS

• Preventing disease transmission through the use of standard precautions is the responsibility of the dental hygienist.

• Work-related risk assessment, engineering controls, and work-practice controls are necessary in reducing occupational exposures.

tuberculosis (TB)

universal precautions

work practice controls
(WPC)

• Ethics play a role in infection-control practices when providing dental hygiene care.

RELEVANCE TO CLINICAL PRACTICE

Dental hygienists may come in contact with communicable diseases when providing dental hygiene care to their patients. It is important for hygienists to understand transmissible diseases and how to prevent their transmission in the dental environment. Previously, dental healthcare personnel (DHCP) followed **universal precautions** that were based on the concept that all blood and body fluids were infectious. In 1996, **standard precautions** were introduced by the Centers for Disease Control and Prevention (CDC) and expanded to include pathogens that can spread by blood or any other body fluid, excretion, or secretion.[1] Standard precautions apply to: (a) contact with blood; (b) all body fluids, secretions, and excretions excluding sweat; (c) nonintact skin; and (d) mucous membranes.[1] Both universal precautions and standard precautions were instituted to protect both DHCP and patients.

The Basics

1. Fill in the missing information.

   The mask should be placed and adjusted before _____ and _____.

   The bendable nosepiece should conform to the _____. The bottom of the mask

   needs to be fully under the _____. Masks should not be worn longer than

   _____ in a wet, heavy aerosol, or spatter environment, no longer than

   _____ in a dry environment. A new mask should be worn for

   _____ being treated. Removal of a mask should be accomplished using bare

   hands and by grasping the _____ rather than touching the contaminated mask.

2. The chest and thigh areas are vulnerable to spatter and aerosols; therefore, an ideal protective covering should cover the clinician's knees.
   A. Both the statement and the reason are correct.
   B. The statement is correct; the reason is incorrect.
   C. Both the statement and the reason are incorrect.
   D. The statement is incorrect; the reason is correct.

3. List the personal protective equipment (PPE) that must be worn by dental health-care providers.

   1) _____

   2) _____

   3) _____

   4) _____

4. According to OSHA, which of the following are examples of engineering controls?
   1) Sharps container
   2) Instrument cassettes
   3) Needle recapping device
   4) One-handed scoop technique
      A. 1 and 2
      B. 3 and 4
      C. 1, 2, and 3
      D. All of the above

5. Which of the following is associated with cytomegalovirus (CMV) disease?
   A. HHV 4
   B. HHV 5
   C. HHV 6
   D. HHV 7
   E. HHV 8

6. Fill in the blanks.

   An infectious agent enters the _____ where the organism lives and multiplies.

   The _____ is the mode of escape such as through saliva and blood. The means

   by which contact occurs is called the _____. The _____ is the

   access site for the agent to pass through the open skin or mucous membrane of the

   _____, which is someone who does not have immunity to the infectious agent.

7. The Organization for Safety and Asepsis Protocol (OSAP) is a nonprofit organization whose mission is:
   A. "to protect human health and the environment."
   B. "to be the world's leading advocate for the safe and infection-free delivery of oral health care."
   C. "protecting consumers and enhancing public health by maximizing compliance of FDA-regulated products and minimizing risk associated with these products."

8. Match the five stages of disease with the corresponding definition.

   _____ Incubation   A. Body begins to heal

   _____ Prodrome   B. Period when infectious agent enters body until symptoms first emerge

   _____ Clinical   C. Symptoms begin to dissipate and patient starts to recover

   _____ Decline   D. Peak of the disease

   _____ Recovery   E. General occurrence of symptoms including fever, nausea, headache

9. Which of the following can only self-replicate in the presence of HBV?
   A. Hepatitis A
   B. Hepatitis C
   C. Hepatitis D
   D. Hepatitis E

Learning Activities

1. Discuss and give examples of direct and indirect modes of transmission.

   _____

   _____

   _____

   _____

2. Review the recommendations for HIV postexposure prophylaxis (PEP) for percutaneous injury.

_____

_____

_____

_____

Board Style Review Questions

1. Which of the following agencies is responsible for developing and enforcing workplace safety and health regulations?
   A. American National Standards Institute (ANSI)
   B. Centers for Disease Control and Prevention (CDC)
   C. National Institute for Occupational Safety and Health (NIOSH)
   D. Occupational Safety and Health Administration (OSHA)

2. All of the following drugs can be used to treat tuberculosis *except* for one. Which one is the *exception?*
   A. Isoniazid (INH)
   B. Rifampin (RIF)
   C. Azidothymidine (AZT)
   D. Ethambutol (EMB)
   E. Pyranzinamide (PZA)

3. Which of the following designates herpes that causes mononucleosis?
   A. HHV 7
   B. HHV 6
   C. HHV 5
   D. HHV 4

4. Herpes simplex 1 (HSV-1) is called herpes labials because it appears on the lips. Infections around the mouth, nose, gingiva, palate, eyes, skin, and the genitals can also manifest.
   A. Both statements are correct.
   B. The first statement is correct; the second statement is incorrect.
   C. Both statements are incorrect.
   D. The first statement is incorrect; the second statement is correct.

5. Herpes simplex 2 (HSV-2) is referred to as genital herpes. It can only be transmitted to the genitalia.
   A. Both statements are correct.
   B. The first statement is correct; the second statement is incorrect.
   C. Both statements are incorrect.
   D. The first statement is incorrect; the second statement is correct.

6. Which of the following drugs is used to treat herpes infections?
   A. Tetracycline
   B. Relenza
   C. Penicillin
   D. Fluconazole
   E. Acyclovir

7. Most individuals infected with this type of hepatitis are unaware of the infection. This type of hepatitis is also considered the most serious form of hepatitis.
   A. Hepatitis A
   B. Hepatitis B
   C. Hepatitis C
   D. Hepatitis D
   E. Hepatitis E

8. Hepatitis A and E are transmitted through contaminated food and water, whereas Hepatitis B, C, and D are transmitted through contact with infectious body fluids.
   A. Both statements are true.
   B. The first statement is true; the second statement is false.
   C. Both statements are false.
   D. The first statement is false; the second statement is true.

9. All of the following statements are correct *except* for one. Which one is the *exception?*
   A. The onset of HIV infection is referred to as AIDS.
   B. HIV is an infection that destroys the immune system.
   C. The diagnosis of AIDS is connected to the development of at least one opportunistic infection.
   D. Of the two types of HIV, HIV-1 is the most common type globally.

10. Aerosols contain droplets of biological contaminants that are greater than 50 µm in diameter. Spatter contains biological contaminants that can be inhaled and are less than 50 µm in diameter.
    A. Both statements are correct.
    B. The first statement is correct; the second is incorrect.
    C. Both statements are incorrect.
    D. The first statement is incorrect; the second statement is correct.

REFERENCES

1. Kohn WG, Collins AS, Cleveland JL, Harte JA, Eklund KJ, Malvitz DM; Centers for Disease Control and Prevention (CDC). Guidelines for infection control in dental health-care settings—2003. *MMWR Recomm Rep.* 2003;52(RR-17):1-61. http://www.cdc.gov/mmwr/preview/mmwrhtml/rr5217a1.htm#top.

Rubric/Process Evaluations

Process Evaluation Template

Infection Control

Evaluation Criteria	Criteria Met? (Y/N)	Comments
Student has hair properly pulled back and secure so as not to fall forward.		
Student wears small earrings only during patient treatment. (Wrist and finger jewelry make it difficult to properly wash hands and place gloves effectively.)		
Nails are short, well manicured.		
Student puts on appropriate protective covering.		
Student dons proper eyewear and provides proper eyewear to patient.		
Fluid-resistant mask with greater than 95% bacterial filtration efficiency (BFE) put on.		
Appropriate hand hygiene measures followed.		
Appropriate gloves donned for procedure.		
Demonstrates proper removal and disposal of contaminated gloves as needed/post procedure.		
Demonstrates proper removal of contaminated mask.		
Student properly disinfects/disposes of contaminated PPE.		
Proper post-treatment hand hygiene performed.		

Part IV

Assessment

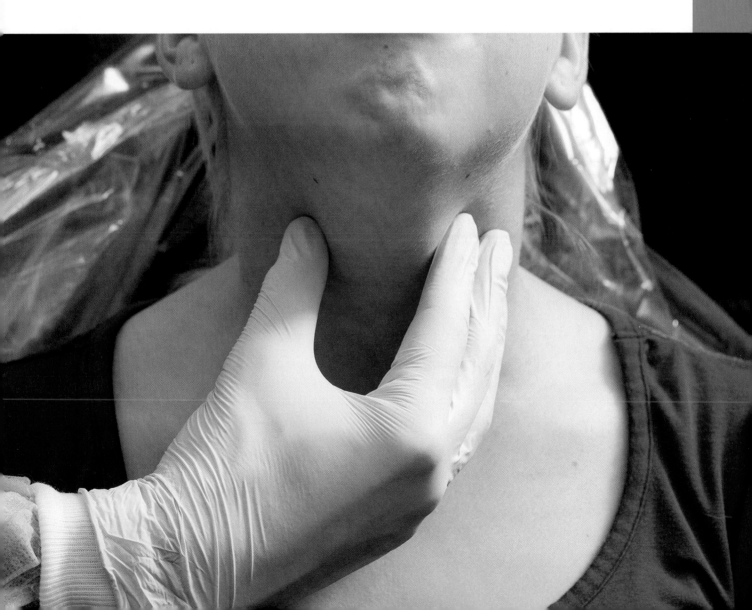

Chapter 8 | Comprehensive Medical and Oral Health History

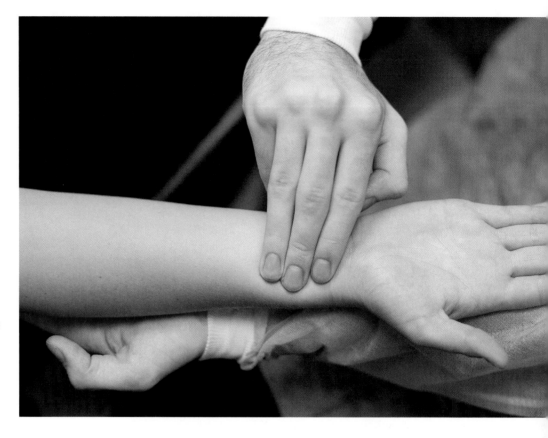

LEARNING OBJECTIVES

After reading this chapter, the student should be able to:

8.1 Identify key components of comprehensive medical and dental histories.

8.2 Use probing questions to elicit accurate information.

8.3 Search sample health histories and customize appropriate to a clinical practice setting.

8.4 Take a comprehensive history and vital signs for each patient.

8.5 Explain the need for a comprehensive and accurate history.

KEY CONCEPTS

• The foundation of patient evaluation and risk assessment is the patient health history.

• Performing a comprehensive health history is vital to determining general and oral health status, determining whether rendering care is appropriate, and avoiding potential medical emergencies.

• As part of the Standards for Clinical Dental Hygiene Practice developed by the American Dental Hygienists' Association, dental hygienists are expected to conduct a thorough assessment of each patient with respect to oral and general health status and patient needs.

• Vital signs are taken at each appointment as a means to identify signs of an infection, as a baseline measure to anticipate and/or prevent a medical emergency, or to identify a diagnosed or undiagnosed systemic condition.

RELEVANCE TO CLINICAL PRACTICE

Every patient who appears for a dental hygiene appointment presents with a unique set of circumstances and physical, mental, social, and emotional health states. Conducting a health history is the first phase of the assessment component of the dental hygiene process of care. Taking the time to perform a comprehensive health history is vital to determining general and oral health status, determining whether rendering care is appropriate, and anticipating potential medical emergencies.

The Basics

1. Bacteremias are more likely caused by dental hygiene procedures than from daily activities. Antibiotic prophylaxis does not always prevent infective endocarditis risk from occurring post invasive oral health care.
   A. Both statements are correct.
   B. Both statements are incorrect.
   C. The first statement is incorrect; the second statement is correct.
   D. The first statement is correct; the second statement is incorrect.

2. Patients often do not remember the name of the medications they are taking, how much they are taking, or for what condition the medication has been prescribed. What measures can be taken to address these potential concerns?

   _____

   _____

   _____

   _____

3. When assessing BMI, normal weight falls under which category?
   A. ≥ 30
   B. 25 to 29.9
   C. 18.5 to 24.9
   D. Less than 18.5

4. List the personal profile information that should be collected during review of the patient history.

   1) _____

   2) _____

   3) _____

   4) _____

   5) _____

   6) _____

5. A normal respiratory rate for children is:
   A. Up to 44 breaths per minute
   B. 14 to 20 breaths per minute
   C. 20 to 24 breaths per minute

6. Recall the elements of the health history.

   1) _____

   2) _____

   3) _____

   4) _____

   5) _____

   6) _____

   7) _____

   8) _____

7. Adequate functional capacity is defined as the individual being able to perform activities that meet a 4 metabolic level of endurance called the 4 metabolic equivalent (MET). A MET is a unit of measure representing the amount of carbon dioxide expelled during physical activity.
   A. Both statements are true.
   B. Both statements are false.
   C. The first statement is true; the second statement is false.
   D. The first statement is false; the second statement is true.

8. List three uses for patient biographical data.

   1) _____

   2) _____

   3) _____

9. Match the following terms with the corresponding definition.

   _____ Bradycardia   A. Difficulty breathing in the supine position

   _____ Dyspnea   B. Slower heart rate of less than 60 bpm

   _____ Hyperventilation   C. Rapid breathing

   _____ Orthopnea   D. Difficulty breathing

   _____ Tachyarrhythmia   E. Fast irregular pulse rate

   _____ Tachycardia   F. Deep, rapid, irregular breathing

   _____ Tachypnea   G. Fast heart rate over 100 bpm in adults

Learning Activities

1. Describe the health history questionnaire developed by the College of Registered Dental Hygienists of Alberta.

   _____

   _____

   _____

   _____

2. Compare and contrast the review of systems-oriented health history to the disease-oriented type of health history.

_____

_____

_____

_____

3. When updating the health history, explain the concerns associated with the question, "Have there been any changes in your health since the last time you were here?"

_____

_____

_____

_____

Board Style Review Questions

1. Select the format that limits dialogue between the patient and the dental hygienist during a patient interview.
   A. Open-ended format
   B. Closed-ended format
   C. Motivational interviewing format
   D. Combination of open-ended and closed-ended formats

2. Which type of patient interview consists of recording the patient's responses on a blank sheet of paper?
   A. Open-ended format
   B. Closed-ended format
   C. Motivational interviewing format
   D. Combination of open-ended and closed-ended formats

3. If a cuff is too small, falsely low values will occur. If a cuff is too large, falsely elevated levels will occur.
   A. Both statements are true.
   B. Both statements are false.

4. A thorough review of personal, medical, oral, and drug histories are used as part of comprehensive dental hygiene care to:
   A. Diagnose systemic conditions
   B. Obtain an informed consent
   C. Anticipate medical emergencies
   D. Identify factors that contribute to general and oral health

5. If the health history must be reviewed in the dental operatory, the dental hygienist should place the patient in the supine position to ensure the patient is comfortable. The dental hygienist and the patient should also be positioned at eye level with each other when discussing health-related questions.
   A. Both statements are correct.
   B. The first statement is correct; the second statement is incorrect.
   C. Both statements are incorrect.
   D. The first statement is incorrect; the second statement is correct.

6. The systems-oriented approach to health histories provides an opportunity to relate signs and symptoms to specific diseases. The signs and symptoms may suggest an undiagnosed condition.
   A. Both statements are correct.
   B. The first statement is correct; the second statement is incorrect.
   C. Both statements are incorrect.
   D. The first statement is incorrect; the second statement is correct.

7. Select the procedures that require antibiotic prophylaxis.
   1) Dental radiographs
   2) Scaling and root planing
   3) Anesthetic injection through noninfected tissue
   4) Routine prophylaxis/debridement
      A. 1 and 2
      B. 2 and 4
      C. 1, 2, and 3
      D. 2, 3, and 4

8. Which one of the following does not require antibiotic prophylaxis?
   A. Palliative shunts
   B. A cardiac transplant that develops a heart valve problem
   C. Artificial heart valves
   D. History of infective endocarditis
   E. A congenital defect repaired with prosthetic material that was completed more than 6 months ago

9. Hypertension is considered:
   1) A systolic blood pressure of 90 mm Hg or higher
   2) A systolic blood pressure of 140 mm Hg or higher
   3) A diastolic blood pressure of 90 mm Hg or higher
   4) A diastolic blood pressure of 140 mm Hg or higher
   5) Taking a medication to reduce blood pressure
      A. 1 and 4
      B. 2 and 3
      C. 1, 4, and 5
      D. 2, 3, and 5
      E. 5 only

10. Your patient has been diagnosed with cancer and presents for his 6 month re-care appointment. All of the following statements are correct for this situation *except* for one. Which one is the *exception?*
    A. Determine whether premedication is indicated.
    B. Check vitals; if they are normal a consult is not necessary, proceed with treatment.
    C. Consult with the oncology team to establish baseline blood assay values.

11. During review of the patient history, the patient reports signs and symptoms suggestive of an undiagnosed systemic condition so the dental hygienist should refer for medical evaluation and diagnostic testing. Second, the hygienist should later call the patient to remind and encourage them to schedule this evaluation.
    A. Both statements are correct.
    B. The first statement is correct; the second is incorrect.
    C. Both statements are incorrect.
    D. The first statement is incorrect; the second statement is correct.

_____

_____

_____

_____

_____

_____

_____

_____

_____

_____

Rubric/Process Evaluation

Process Evaluation Template

Health History Review

Evaluation Criteria	Criteria Met? (Y/N)	Comments
Student collected pertinent biographical data (name, address, phone, e-mail, date of birth, sex, ethnicity, marital status, occupation).		
Student reviewed physician's name and contact information with patient.		
Chief complaint of chief concern was addressed and recorded.		
General health including family history was reviewed.		
Oral/dental history reviewed.		
Personal psychosocial history reviewed.		
Medication history.		
Vital signs assessed (temperature, pulse, respiration, blood pressure).		
Height, weight, BMI recorded.		
Evidence of critical thinking/decision-making by student after review of histories (physician referral, consultation, determination of premedication requirements, etc.).		
Student conducted a thorough patient interview using appropriate probing questions to elicit accurate information.		
Patient interview conducted in an appropriate setting. Patient seated upright and at eye level to student.		

Chapter 9 | Assessment Instruments

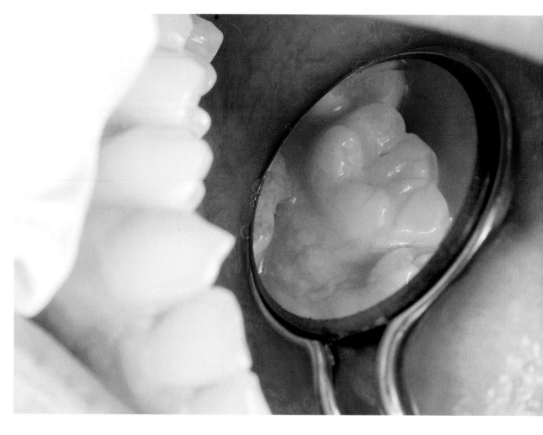

LEARNING OBJECTIVES

After reading this chapter, the student should be able to:

9.1 Describe the different types of assessment instruments.

9.2 Outline different types of mirrors, explorers, and probes and their uses.

9.3 Properly activate all assessment instruments.

9.4 Demonstrate correct technique in using assessment instruments.

KEY CONCEPTS

• Assessment instruments are essential tools used for dental hygiene care.

• There are numerous varieties and types of assessment instruments.

• Different types of instruments are better suited for certain purposes.

RELEVANCE TO CLINICAL PRACTICE

Assessment is a key step in providing optimal dental hygiene care to patients. **Assessment** can be defined as "the process of gathering information from the patient relative to general health and oral health status, medical history, medications, current needs and concerns."[1] The American Dental Hygienists' Association includes assessment in the Standards for Clinical Dental Hygiene Practice, a guide and expectation of the role dental hygienists play in the treatment of patients.[2] Being able to accurately and thoroughly complete assessments is an essential skill a dental hygienist must have. Assessments help to guide treatment options and help dental hygienists and patients make choices to obtain optimal oral health. In 2007 it was reported that dental hygienists spend 11.2 hours per week doing dental hygiene assessments, third to prophylaxis (21.4 hours) and patient education (11.8 hours).[3] This chapter discusses the basic instruments necessary to complete a clinical assessment. Other chapters within this textbook focus on periodontal, risk, nutritional, and caries assessments.

The Basics

1. Which assessment instrument allows the dental hygienist to use tactile sensitivity?
    A. Explorer
    B. Furcation probe
    C. Mirror
    D. Periodontal probe

2. Indirect vision is:
    A. Used to reflect light onto intraoral surfaces.
    B. Used to direct light off the mirror through the anterior teeth.
    C. Used to create a magnified image.
    D. Used with a dental mirror to view an intraoral structure that cannot be seen directly.

3. Explorers with lightweight handles allow for better sensitivity. The shank and working ends are thin and flexible to allow vibrations to be carried to the clinician's fingers.
    A. Both statements are true.
    B. The first statement is true; the second statement is false.
    C. Both statements are false.
    D. The first statement is false; the second statement is true.

4. What is (are) the insertion site(s) for the furcation probe on the maxillary molars?
    1) Distolingual
    2) Mesiobuccal
    3) Mesiolingual
    4) Midbuccal
        A. 1 and 3
        B. 1, 2, and 3
        C. 1, 3, and 4
        D. 2, 3, and 4

5. Which mirror surface provides a clear, undistorted image?
   A. Concave
   B. Curved
   C. Front
   D. Plane

6. Using your finger for retraction is most comfortable for the patient, but using the mirror to retract tissue can be done comfortably. Most commonly, the mirror is held in the clinician's nondominant hand and used for retraction of the tongue and the buccal mucosa.
   A. Both statements are correct.
   B. The first statement is correct; the second statement is incorrect.
   C. Both statements are incorrect.
   D. The first statement is incorrect; the second statement is correct.

7. The periodontal probe can be used for all of the following *except* one. Which one is the *exception?*
   A. Measuring clinical attachment loss.
   B. Examining tooth anatomy.
   C. Measuring the width of attached gingiva.
   D. Measuring the size of oral lesions.

8. Which type of mirror surface creates a magnified image?
   A. Flat
   B. Front
   C. Curved
   D. Plane

9. The pigtail explorer can be used for:
   A. Supragingival examination of caries
   B. Calculus detection in deep pockets
   C. Examination of margins of restorations
   D. Calculus detection in healthy pockets

10. Identify the mirror surface that provides a double-image.
    A. Concave
    B. Curved
    C. Front
    D. Plane

Learning Activities

1. Explain how scratching the face of the mirror can be prevented during ultrasonic cleaning and autoclaving.

_____

_____

_____

_____

_____

_____

_____

_____

_____

_____

_____

_____

2. Practice activating the assessment instruments on a typodont. Have a student partner provide a peer-evaluation of your technique.

_____

_____

_____

_____

_____

_____

_____

_____

_____

_____

_____

_____

3. Research the various technologies (e.g., Florida Probe) available that can be used to improve the efficiency of completing assessments. What are the benefits and limitations of these technologies?

_____

_____

_____

_____

_____

_____

_____

_____

_____

_____

_____

_____

Board Style Review Questions

1. Select the statement that best describes the advantage of using a double-sided mirror.
   A. It allows for safe insertion into the oral cavity.
   B. It rotates for better visualization.
   C. It is convenient and more ergonomic than a single-sided mirror.
   D. It is lightweight.

2. The Shepherd's Hook explorer is best used for:
   A. Subgingival calculus detection
   B. Caries detection
   C. Root surface exploration
   D. Root caries detection

3. Where should the middle finger of the dominant hand rest on an explorer?
   A. Handle
   B. Mirror head
   C. Shank
   D. Working end

4. Which explorer is best used for calculus detection in healthy pockets but not for deep pockets?
   A. Pigtail
   B. Shepherd's Hook
   C. Straight
   D. 11/12

5. If the dental hygienist has difficulty viewing the intraoral surfaces because it is too dark, the clinician can use:
   A. Direct vision
   B. Illumination
   C. Modified pen grasp
   D. Retraction

6. The insertion site(s) for the furcation probe on mandibular molars is(are):
   A. Mesiolingual
   B. Midbuccal
   C. Midbuccal, distolingual, mesiolingual
   D. Midbuccal, midlingual

7. As the probe is moved into the proximal surface, the dental hygienist should:
   A. Apply more pressure.
   B. Remove the probe from the sulcus.
   C. Make sure the probe tip is away from the tooth.
   D. Slant the probe so it reaches under the contact area.

8. All of the following statements are correct of the explorer *except* for one. Which one is the *exception?*
   A. Light overlapping, vertical, horizontal, and oblique strokes should be used.
   B. The shank and working ends allow vibrations to be carried to the clinician's fingers.
   C. Only wrist activation is acceptable to use with the explorer.
   D. The sides of the tip are used to detect calculus and surface irregularities.

9. The clinician must select the proper working end of the furcation probe. The terminal shank should be positioned parallel to the tooth surface.
   A. Both statements are true.
   B. The first statement is true; the second statement is false.
   C. Both statements are false.
   D. The first statement is false; the second statement is true.

10. The periodontal probe may be used for all of the following *except* for one. Which one is the *exception?*
    A. Evaluating furcations on multirooted teeth.
    B. Measuring clinical attachment loss.
    C. Measuring the size of oral lesions.
    D. Assessing the presence of purulence.

Active Learning

For each of these exercises, reference the photograph following the question.

1. Is this the correct or incorrect working end? Circle the answer.

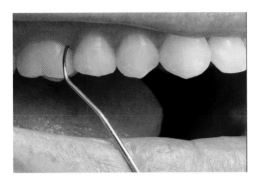

Correct   Incorrect
Explain your rationale:

_____

_____

_____

_____

_____

_____

2. Is the modified pen grasp correct or incorrect?

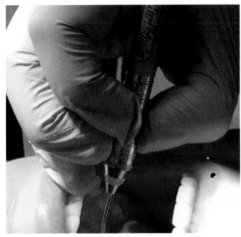

Correct   Incorrect
Explain your rationale:

_____

_____

_____

_____

_____

_____

3. How could this modified pen grasp be improved?

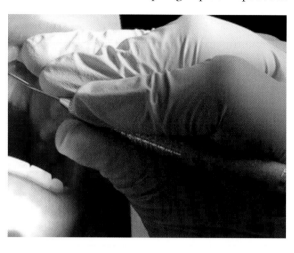

_____

_____

_____

_____

_____

_____

4. Is this the correct or incorrect working end for the Naber's furcation probe?
   Correct   Incorrect

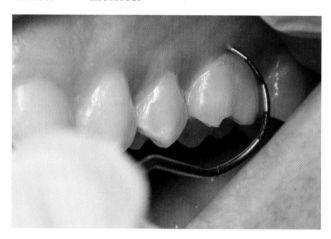

REFERENCES

1. Gibson-Howell J, Hicks M. Dental hygienists' role in patient assessments and clinical examinations in U.S. dental practices: a review of the literature. *J Allied Health.* 2010;39(1):e1-e5.
2. American Dental Hygienists' Association. Standards for clinical dental hygiene practice. March 10, 2008. Available from: http://www.adha.org/downloads/adha_standards08.pdf. Accessed February 12, 2010.
3. American Dental Hygienists' Association. Survey of dental hygienists in the United States, 2007: executive summary. 2009. Available from: http://www.adha.org/downloads/DH_practitioner_survey_Exec_Summary.pdf. Accessed on March 1, 2010.

Rubrics/Process Evaluations

Process Evaluation Template

Explorer

Evaluation Criteria	Criteria Met? (Y/N)	Comments
The student. . .		
Properly positions the patient.		
Selects the proper end of the explorer.		
Uses a light, modified pen grasp with middle finger resting on the shank.		
Establishes an appropriate fulcrum.		
Keeps the last 1 to 2 mm of the tip adapted to the tooth surface.		
Rolls the instrument handle between index finger and thumb to maintain adaptation and keep terminal shank parallel with the long axis of the tooth.		
Uses light overlapping, vertical, horizontal, and oblique strokes.		
Inserts the tip to the base of the pocket.		
Uses exploratory strokes before, during, and after scaling.		
Uses standard precautions during procedure.		

Rubrics/Process Evaluations

Process Evaluation Template

Periodontal Probe

Evaluation Criteria	Criteria Met? (Y/N)	Comments
The student. . .		
Properly positions the patient.		
Uses a light, modified pen grasp.		
Establishes an appropriate fulcrum.		
Keeps the probe tip against the tooth.		
Probe is kept parallel to the long axis except when adapting to the proximal surfaces.		
Uses a walking stroke that is 1 to 2 mm vertical and 1 mm horizontal.		
Does not remove the probe from the sulcus until moving to the next tooth.		
Uses light pressure. Wrist or digital activation is acceptable.		
As the probe is moved into the proximal surface, it is slanted to reach the contact area.		
Uses standard precautions during procedure.		

Chapter 10 | Extraoral and Intraoral Examination

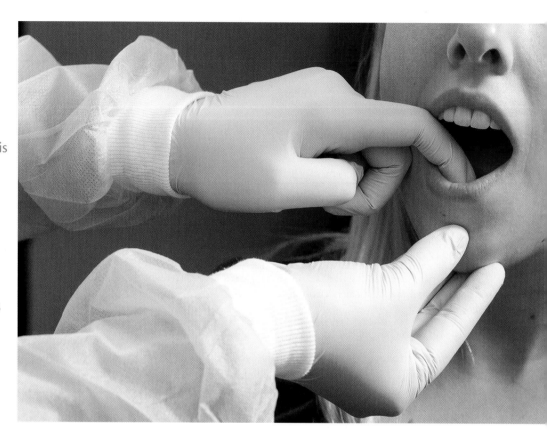

LEARNING OBJECTIVES

After reading this chapter, the student should be able to:

10.1 Perform a thorough, standardized extraoral and intraoral examination.

10.2 Identify clinical signs and symptoms of oral diseases and oral manifestations of systemic diseases.

10.3 Demonstrate a working knowledge of the language of oral pathology and an understanding of the etiology, pathogenesis, and structural and functional deviations resulting from the disease process.

10.4 Describe findings.

10.5 Select, obtain, and interpret information using a variety of diagnostic procedures consistent with medico-legal principles.

10.6 Develop a differential diagnosis derived from collected data consistent with medico-legal principles.

10.7 Recognize predisposing and causative risk factors requiring intervention to prevent disease.

10.8 Discuss findings with dental and other health-care professionals, as well as with the patient, according to the standards of evidence-based dental hygiene care.

incisional biopsy

induration

inflammatory fibrous hyperplasia

inflammatory papillary hyperplasia

in situ

irritation fibroma

leukoedema

leukoplakia

linea alba

mandibular torus

metastasis

oral and maxillofacial pathology

palatal torus

paresthesia

peripheral giant cell granuloma

peripheral ossifying fibroma (POF)

pregnancy tumor

pyogenic granuloma

reactive conditions

speckled leukoplakia

squamous cell carcinoma

staging

tissue autofluorescence

tissue reflectance

toluidine blue dye

torus mandibularis

torus palatinus

traumatic fibroma

tumor board

vital tissue staining technology

wandering rash of the tongue

10.9 Explain how to use a variety of tools for early detection of oral cancer.

10.10 Make appropriate referrals for evidence-based care.

10.11 Use evidence-based decision-making to appraise and integrate emerging treatment modalities.

KEY CONCEPTS

- Knowledge of normal head and neck anatomy as well as skills necessary to perform a complete assessment of head and neck structures (extraoral and intraoral examination and oral cancer screening) are paramount to the early detection of head and neck abnormalities.
- Squamous cell carcinoma is the most common malignancy of the oral cavity. Knowledge of the cause, development, prevalence, risk factors, and characteristics of *all* oral lesions and pathology is critical in the development of a differential diagnosis.
- Developmental conditions may be congenital (present at birth) or may develop later in life, but once they have developed they are nonprogressive. They often require no intervention unless they interfere with normal function or esthetics.
- Reactive conditions occur in response to some type of environmental factor such as trauma. Underlying causes of these findings must be addressed to prevent recurrence.
- There are a number of commercial adjunctive techniques for detecting oral cancer, including vital tissue staining, visualization adjuncts, and exfoliative cytology (brush test); however, current dental literature has not provided evidence that they detect oral cancer earlier.
- The gold standard for a **definitive diagnosis** of any finding is the biopsy: an incisional biopsy for large lesions or lesions that are suspected to be cancerous, or both; and an excisional biopsy for small or harmless-appearing lesions, or both.

RELEVANCE TO CLINICAL PRACTICE

Published studies show that currently less than 15% of those who visit a dentist regularly report having had an oral cancer screening.[1] This is unfortunate when the greatest strides in combating most cancers have come from increased awareness and aggressive campaigns directed at early detection. Cancers of the head and neck, which include cancers of the oral cavity, larynx, pharynx, thyroid, salivary glands, and nose/nasal passages, account for approximately 6% of all malignancies in the United States.[2] An estimated 28,500 new cases (20,100 male and 8,400 female cases) of oral cavity and oropharyngeal cancer were diagnosed in 2009.[3,4] An estimated 6,100 people (4,200 male and 1,900 female individuals) will die of these cancers.[3]

Oftentimes the dental profession is the first line of defense in early detection of head and neck abnormalities including, but not limited to, head and neck cancer. One of the roles of a dental professional is to perform an examination of the head and neck region to recognize deviations from normal anatomy and structures so that proper referral to the appropriate health-care professional can be made if necessary.

The procedures and techniques involved with the extraoral and intraoral (head and neck) examination will be presented in this chapter. A discussion of oral lesions and pathology will serve as a foundation for recognizing variations from normal structures. Normal anatomy will be highlighted by way of photos and illustrations. A discussion on the manner in which this examination serves as an oral cancer screening as well as a tool for oral cancer prevention will also be provided.

The Basics

1. When detecting oral cancer clinically, the clinician should recognize the following warning signs of change. Which of these is least likely to be a warning sign of cancer?
   A. Nonhealing extraction site
   B. Lymph nodes may feel firm, fixed, and enlarged on palpation
   C. Persistent hoarse voice
   D. Persistent ulcerations that heal within 2 weeks

2. Leukoedema appears clinically as:
   A. A grayish-white opalescence that does not change when stretched.
   B. A grayish-white opalescence that disappears when stretched.
   C. A condition seen unilaterally on the buccal mucosa.
   D. A condition that requires excisional biopsy.

3. List the components that should be included for thorough documentation of intraoral lesions.

   1) _____

   2) _____

   3) _____

   4) _____

   5) _____

4. The cause of dysplastic transformation of oral epithelium is the development of specific genetic mutations most strongly linked to tobacco use. The risk of developing oral cavity and oropharyngeal cancer increases with the amount of tobacco smoked or chewed.
   A. Both statements are correct.
   B. The first statement is correct; the second statement is incorrect.
   C. Both statements are incorrect.
   D. The first statement is incorrect; the second statement is correct.

5. A thickened white line in response to friction is termed:
   A. Epulis
   B. Fibroma
   C. Linea alba
   D. Leukoedema

6. A lesion that occurs in the vestibular mucosa and appears as folds of fibrous tissue is referred to as:
   A. Peripheral giant cell granuloma
   B. Pyogenic granuloma
   C. Epulis fissuratum
   D. Fissured tongue

7. All of the following describe gingival fibromatosis *except* for one. Which one is the *exception?*
   A. It is frequently drug-induced.
   B. It is often aggravated by poor oral hygiene.
   C. Localized enlargement of the gingiva.
   D. Lesions are surgically excised.

8. Purple dome-shaped nodules are called:
   A. Papillary hyperplasia
   B. Peripheral giant cell granuloma
   C. Peripheral ossifying fibroma
   D. Palatal torus

9. Choose the condition that is most commonly found in the anterior maxillary arch.
   A. Benign migratory glossitis
   B. Fibroma
   C. Papillary hyperplasia
   D. Peripheral ossifying fibroma

Learning Activities

1. Discuss the objectives of performing an extraoral and intraoral examination.

   _____

   _____

   _____

   _____

2. Choose a diagnostic tool for oral cancer. Explain the technique for using the tool. Describe the benefits and challenges to using this tool.

   _____

   _____

   _____

   _____

Board Style Review Questions

1. Which type of biopsy involves the complete removal of a lesion for diagnosis?
   A. Cytological smear
   B. Excisional
   C. Incisional
   D. Punch

2. The most common sites for oral squamous cell carcinoma are the:
   1) Lateral or ventral surfaces of the tongue
   2) Dorsal surface of the tongue
   3) Floor of the mouth
   4) Buccal mucosa
      A. 1 and 3
      B. 1 and 4
      C. 2 and 3
      D. 2 and 4

3. Choose the condition that occurs when the filiform papilla become abnormally elongated.
   A. Gingival epulis
   B. Gingival fibromatosis
   C. Hairy tongue
   D. Papillary hyperplasia

4. Palpable nodes arising from acute inflammatory conditions tend to be fixed, nontender, and hard. Palpable nodes due to malignant disease tend to be freely movable and tender.
   A. Both statements are correct.
   B. The first statement is correct; the second statement is incorrect.
   C. Both statements are incorrect.
   D. The first statement is incorrect; the second statement is correct.

5. Which of these conditions can result in halitosis or irritation from food debris accumulations?
   A. Epulis fissuratum
   B. Exostosis
   C. Fissured tongue
   D. Fordyce granules

6. The term pedunculated refers to:
   A. Benign tumor-like growth
   B. Attached directly
   C. Blood vessel proliferation
   D. Attached by an elongated stalk of tissue

7. A biopsy must be performed with a lesion that appears as well delineated and red with a velvety surface texture. Which lesion does this describe?
   A. Erythroplakia
   B. Leukoplakia
   C. Leukoedema
   D. Fibroma

8. Hepatitis A and E are transmitted through contaminated food and water, whereas hepatitis B, C, and D are transmitted through contact with infectious body fluids.
   A. Both statements are true.
   B. The first statement is true; the second statement is false.
   C. Both statements are false.
   D. The first statement is false; the second statement is true.

9. All of the following characteristics can be used to assess the tissue when clinically identifying oral cancer except for one. Which one is the exception?
   A. Color
   B. Consistency
   C. Contour
   D. Function
   E. Sensation

10. Which of the following is the most common benign tumor-like growth in the oral cavity?
    A. Fibroma
    B. Gingival fibromatosis
    C. Linea alba
    D. Papillary hyperplasia

Active Learning

Match the photos to the corresponding terminology.

1. _____

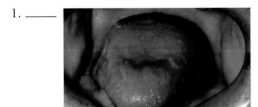

Photo courtesy of Phillip Dunn, DDS

A. Ankyloglossia

2. _____

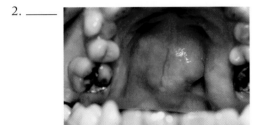

Photo courtesy of Phillip Dunn, DDS

B. Erythroplakia

3. _____

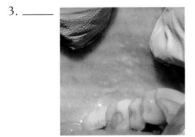

Photo provided by Tammy Sanderson

C. Fissured tongue

4. _____

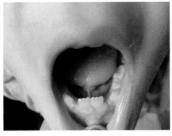

Photo courtesy of Nicole Uhl, RDH

D. Forydyce granules

5. _____

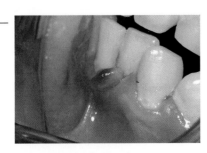

Photo courtesy of Phillip Dunn, DDS

E. Geographic tongue

6. _____

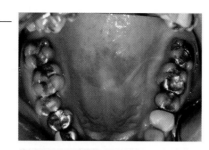

Photo courtesy of Phillip Dunn, DDS

F. Leukoplakia

7. _____

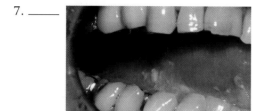

Photo courtesy of Phillip Dunn, DDS

G. Pyogenic granuloma

8. _____

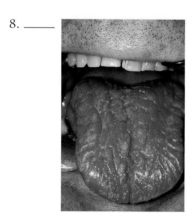

Photo courtesy of Phillip Dunn, DDS

H. Torus palatinus

REFERENCES

1. Oral Cancer Foundation. The role of dental and medical professionals. http://www.oralcancerfoundation.org/dental/role_of_dentists.htm. Modified March 2014. Accessed June 9, 2010.
2. National Cancer Institute. Oral cancer screening PDQ. http://www.cancer.gov/cancertopics/pdq/screening/oral/HealthProfessional/page3. Accessed June 9, 2010.
3. National Cancer Institute. A snapshot of head and neck cancers. http://www.cancer.gov/aboutnci/servingpeople/snapshots/head-neck.pdf. Accessed June 9, 2010.
4. American Cancer Society. Detailed guide: oral cavity and oropharyngeal cancer. http://www.cancer.org/docroot/CRI/content/CRI_2_4_1X_What_is_oral_cavity_and_oropharyngeal_cancer_60.asp?rnav=cri. Accessed June 1, 2010.

Rubrics/Process Evaluations

Process Evaluation Template		
Extraoral and Intraoral Examination		
Evaluation Criteria	**Criteria Met? (Y/N)**	**Comments**
Student has necessary armamentarium (gauze, mouth mirror, etc.).		
Student examines the face, skin, voice, nose, eyes, and lips.		
Student performs bilateral palpation of TMJ.		
Palpates auricular regions.		
Palpates parotic region.		
Palpates the submandibular triangle.		
Palpates the submental triangle region.		
Palpates the anterior midline.		
Palpates the sternocleidomastoid muscle.		
Palpates the deep and superficial cervical lymph nodes.		
Palpates supraclavicular nodes.		
Palpates posterior triangles.		
Visually inspects the oral cavity.		
Palpates lips and labial mucosa.		
Inspects and palpates buccal mucosa.		
Inspects gingiva.		
Inspects and palpates tongue and floor of mouth.		
Inspects tonsillar/pharyngeal region.		
Inspects and palpates palate.		
Inspects and palpates alveolar ridge.		
Student uses standard precautions during procedure.		

Chapter 11 | The Periodontal Examination

KEY TERMS

acute inflammation

alveolar bone proper

alveoli

attached gingiva

bleeding on probing
(BOP)

cementoenamel
junction (CEJ)

chronic inflammation

clinical attachment
level (CAL)

col

collagen

exudate

free gingiva

fremitus

furcation

gingival crevicular fluid

gingival recession

gingival sulcus

gingivitis

inflammation

mucogingival junction

papilla

periodontal disease

periodontal risk
assessment

periodontal screening
and recording (PSR)

periodontitis

periodontium

probe depth

refractory

suppuration

tooth mobility

LEARNING OBJECTIVES

After reading this chapter, the student should be able to:

11.1 Describe the tissues of the periodontium.

11.2 State the difference between the periodontal screening and recording
(PSR) and a comprehensive periodontal examination.

11.3 List and describe how to assess each component of a comprehensive
periodontal examination.

11.4 Satisfactorily perform each of the components of a comprehensive
periodontal examination.

11.5 Identify the clinical signs and symptoms of periodontal disease.

11.6 Recognize radiographic findings of periodontal disease.

11.7 Review current systems of classifications of periodontal diseases.

11.8 Accurately record the data collected during the periodontal examination.

KEY CONCEPTS

• A thorough assessment of the periodontium must be conducted to arrive at
an accurate dental hygiene diagnosis, plan appropriate treatment,
implement appropriate treatment, and adequately evaluate treatment
outcomes.

- Periodontal diseases are a group of diseases typically characterized by bacterial infection of the periodontium. Although the initial bacterial challenge to a susceptible host begins with a local inflammatory reaction, most of the damage to the periodontium is due to the host's immune response to the predominantly gram-negative microorganisms.
- Radiographic assessment of the periodontium must accompany a periodontal examination because a periodontal diagnosis should be derived from a combination of sources.
- Adjunctive techniques such as microbial testing, gingival crevicular fluid assays, subgingival temperature, and/or genetic testing may be useful in risk assessment and screening.
- The American Academy of Periodontology (AAP) classification of periodontal diseases provides a general framework for studying the cause, pathogenesis, and treatment of periodontal diseases.

RELEVANCE TO CLINICAL PRACTICE

A thorough periodontal assessment includes evaluation of all aspects of the **periodontium** for signs of inflammation and resultant damage. Together with the medical and dental histories, extraoral and intraoral examination, and dental assessment, the periodontal assessment contributes to the comprehensive data required for diagnosis and treatment planning, as well as a basis for determining treatment plans and outcomes, subsequent treatment needs, and long-term monitoring of oral health.[1-3] The purpose of this chapter is to provide an overview of periodontal anatomy, itemize and describe the components of the comprehensive periodontal examination, and review the American Academy of Periodontology (AAP) classifications of **periodontal diseases** and conditions.[4]

The Basics

1. The term **sulcus** implies an increased probing depth due to apical migration of the junctional epithelium or from gingival inflammation. The term **pocket** defines the space between the tooth and the free gingiva.
    A. Both statements are correct.
    B. The first statement is correct; the second statement is incorrect.
    C. Both statements are incorrect.
    D. The first statement is incorrect; the second statement is correct.

2. The attachment apparatus includes all of the following *except* one. Which one is the *exception?*
    A. Dentin
    B. Periodontal ligament
    C. Alveolar bone
    D. Cementum

3. The free gingiva:
    A. Is nonkeratinized
    B. Is attached by gingival fibers
    C. Forms the outer soft tissue wall of the gingival sulcus
    D. Tapers to meet the tooth and is described as blunted

4. Acutely inflamed gingiva typically appears:
   A. Pink
   B. Red
   C. Coral pink
   D. Bluish

5. The consistency of the gingival tissue in health is:
   A. Rounded or rolled
   B. Scalloped and knife-edged
   C. Soft or spongy
   D. Firm and resilient

6. List the assessment criteria used for a gingival description.

   1) _____

   _____

   _____

   2) _____

   _____

   _____

   3) _____

   _____

   _____

   4) _____

   _____

   _____

7. Identify the incorrect statement.
   A. Periodontitis is inflammation of the structures of the periodontium.
   B. Gingivitis is localized inflammation with apical migration of the junctional epithelium.
   C. Periodontitis begins as gingivitis.
   D. Not all gingivitis progresses to periodontitis.

8. List the primary functions of collagen fibers.

   1) _____

   _____

   _____

   2) _____

   _____

   _____

   3) _____

   _____

   _____

9. Place a "K" next to the keratinized areas of the oral mucosa and an "N" next to the nonkeratinized areas of the oral mucosa.

_____ Labial aspect of the free gingiva

_____ Ventral of the tongue

_____ Soft palate

_____ Alveolar, buccal, and labial mucosa

_____ Hard palate

_____ Junctional epithelium

_____ Attached gingiva

_____ Floor of the mouth

10. Which type of gingival fibers form around the supracrestal portion of an implant?
    A. Circular
    B. Dentogingival
    C. Alveologingival
    D. Dentoperiosteal

Learning Activities

1. Explain how to assess for fremitus.

_____

_____

_____

_____

_____

_____

2. Discuss local risk factors that may contribute to periodontal disease.

_____

_____

_____

_____

_____

_____

3. Create an oral presentation on a periodontal adjunctive technique (microbial testing, biochemical assays, etc.).

_____

_____

_____

_____

_____

_____

_____

_____

Board Style Review Questions

1. Furcation involvement should be suspected when the loss of clinical attachment level (CAL) is:
   A. 3 mm
   B. 4 mm
   C. 5 mm
   D. 6 mm

2. All of the following are associated with the junctional epithelium *except* for one. Which one is the *exception?*
   A. Thick
   B. Nonkeratinized
   C. Base of the sulcus
   D. Attaches the gingiva to the tooth surface

3. The extent or distribution of periodontal disease is classified as localized or generalized. What percentage of sites must be involved for a case to be classified as generalized?
   A. Greater than 20%
   B. Greater than 30%
   C. Greater than 50%
   D. Greater than 65%

4. Which of these does not comprise lamina propria?
   A. Ground substance
   B. Collagen fibers
   C. Osteoblasts
   D. Fibroblasts

5. Keratinized epithelial cells have no nuclei and are stronger than nonkeratinized epithelium. Nonkeratinized epithelial cells are more flexible and have nuclei.
   A. Both statements are correct.
   B. The first statement is correct; the second statement is incorrect.
   C. Both statements are incorrect.
   D. The first statement is incorrect; the second statement is correct.

6. A code of 3 in a single sextant for the Periodontal Screening and Recording (PSR) indicates:
   A. Probing depth of greater than 5.5 mm
   B. The need for a complete periodontal probing of that sextant
   C. Gingival tissues are healthy with no bleeding
   D. Clinical abnormalities such as furcation invasion and mobility

7. Which of these is not considered a principal gingival fiber group?
   A. Circular
   B. Dentogingival
   C. Semicircular
   D. Transseptal

8. A grade III furcation is described as:
   A. Incipient bone loss in the furcation area
   B. Complete bone loss resulting in a through-and-through opening in the furcation
   C. Allow the furcation opening to be visualized
   D. Partial bone loss producing a cul-de-sac

9. Use the following table to answer question 9. For the measurement of #30 D, the clinical attachment level is:
   A. 1 mm
   B. 3 mm
   C. 5 mm
   D. 7 mm

10. Use the following table to answer question 10. The gingival margin for #30 F is:
    A. Apical to the cementoenamel junction
    B. Coronal to the cementoenamel junction
    C. At or slightly coronal to the cementoenamel junction

		#30	
	D	F	M
Probe Depth	4	3	4
Gingival Margin	-1	0	-1
CAL			

Active Learning

Use the radiographs to answer questions 1 to 3.

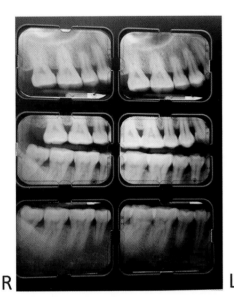

R   L

1. Refer to the posterior bitewing radiograph. Determine the periodontal classification for this patient.
    A. Gingivitis
    B. Slight chronic periodontitis
    C. Moderate chronic periodontitis
    D. Severe chronic periodontitis

2. The extent of bone loss for this patient is classified as:
    A. Generalized horizontal bone loss
    B. Generalized vertical bone loss
    C. Localized horizontal bone loss
    D. No bone loss evident

3. A PSR assessment was performed on this patient. What are the limitations of this assessment?
   1) Millimeter readings are not recorded.
   2) Evaluation of all aspects of the periodontium is not recorded.
   3) Gingival description is not recorded.
   4) Bleeding sites are not recorded.
      A. 1 and 2
      B. 2 and 3
      C. 1, 3, and 4
      D. 1, 2, 3, and 4

Use the following photograph to answer the following questions.

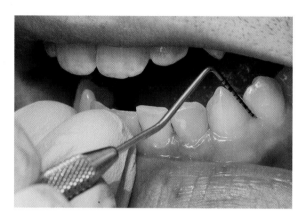

4. What is the correct periodontal measurement for #21M?
   A. 1 mm
   B. 2 mm
   C. 3 mm
   D. 4 mm

5. Select the best gingival description for the tissue in the photograph.
   A. Pink, firm, rolled, shiny
   B. Pale pink, scalloped, firm
   C. Pale pink, knife-edged, firm, shiny
   D. Pink, blunted, firm, shiny

REFERENCES

1. American Academy of Periodontology. Position paper: diagnosis of periodontal diseases. *J Periodontal.* 2003;74(8):1237-1247.
2. American Academy of Periodontology. Position paper: guidelines for periodontal therapy. *J Periodontal.* 2001;72(11):1624-1628.
3. Armitage GC. The complete periodontal examination. *Periodontol 2000.* 2004;34:22-33.
4. Armitage GC. Development of a classification system for periodontal diseases and conditions. *Ann Periodontal.* 1999;4:1-6.

Rubrics/Process Evaluations

Process Evaluation Template		
Periodontal Assessment		
Evaluation Criteria	**Criteria Met? (Y/N)**	**Comments**
Student provides a gingival description that includes color, contour, consistency, and texture.		
Student assesses probe depths within 1 mm of instructor.		
Student records bleeding on probing.		
Student records the level of the free gingiva.		
Student determines the clinical attachment level (CAL).		
Student detects furcation involvement.		
Student identifies suppuration, mobility, and fremitus.		
Student evaluates mucogingival involvement.		
Student completes peri-implant assessment if applicable.		
Oral hygiene assessment completed.		
Student recognizes contributing local and systemic factors.		
Student uses standard precautions during procedure.		
Student completes appropriate documentation.		
Student educates patient about periodontal examination findings.		

Chapter 12 | Hard Tissue Examination

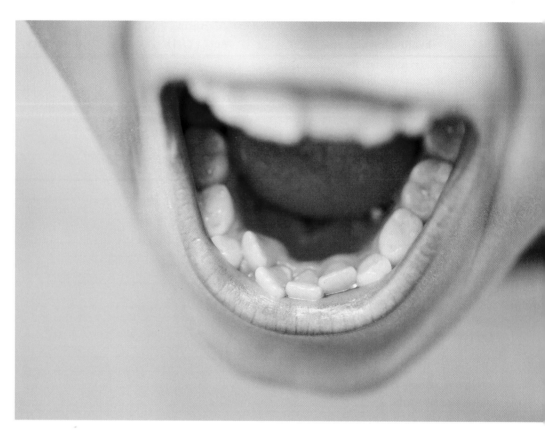

LEARNING OBJECTIVES

After reading this chapter, the student should be able to:

12.1 Assign the correct tooth designation using the appropriate numbering system.

12.2 Identify and chart normal and abnormal conditions of the dentition.

12.3 Properly classify the occlusion according to the Angles Classification of occlusion.

12.4 Recognize new technology in the identification of carious lesions.

KEY CONCEPTS

- Accurate dental charting is an essential role of the dental hygienist.
- Teeth can be identified using a variety of numbering systems.
- Caries can be classified using a standard classification system.
- Dentitions can be classified using the Angle classification of occlusion.
- New technology exists to aid in the early detection of carious lesions.

RELEVANCE TO CLINICAL PRACTICE

Documenting an accurate record of the dentition is an integral part of the patient assessment process. The dental hygienist is often responsible for completing a dental chart at the initial patient visit and updating it on subsequent visits. A current and accurate dental chart is important for the quality planning of dental care, communication with other professions, legal documentation of dental treatment procedures, and forensics.

The Basics

1. Palmer's notation is a system in which a right angle symbol designates each quadrant. In this system, the numbers used to identify the teeth in the maxillary arch are 1 to 16 and the mandibular arch is assigned numbers 17 to 32.
   A. Both statements are correct.
   B. Both statements are incorrect.
   C. The first statement is incorrect; the second statement is correct.
   D. The first statement is correct; the second statement is incorrect.

2. Explain how to measure the amount of overbite.

   _____

   _____

   _____

   _____

   _____

   _____

3. In the Universal Numbering System, the tooth numbers for the maxillary and mandibular first premolars are:
   A. #2, 15, 18, 31
   B. #4, 13, 20, 29
   C. #5, 12, 20, 29
   D. #5, 12, 21, 28

4. Define the following terms that relate to malpositioned individual teeth.

   1) Buccoversion: _____

   _____

   2) Labioversion: _____

   _____

   3) Linguoversion: _____

   _____

   4) Supraversion: _____

   _____

   5) Infraversion: _____

   _____

   6) Torsoversion: _____

   _____

5. In the Universal Numbering System, the primary canines are designated as:
   A. 53, 63, 73, 83
   B. c, h, m, r
   C. 6, 11, 22, 27
   D. 13, 23, 33, 43
   E. d, g, n, q

6. The normal or desired occlusion of the primary dentition is referred to as:
   A. Crossbite
   B. Distal step
   C. Mesial step
   D. Terminal plane

7. In the Universal Numbering System, the primary maxillary right second molar is identified as letter "A". The primary second molar in the mandibular right quadrant is identified as "T".
   A. Both statements are true.
   B. Both statements are false.
   C. The first statement is true; the second statement is false.
   D. The first statement is false; the second statement is true

8. List four reasons why it is important to maintain a current and accurate dental chart.

   1) _____

      _____

      _____

   2) _____

      _____

      _____

   3) _____

      _____

      _____

   4) _____

      _____

      _____

9. Match the following G.V. Black Classification terms with the corresponding definition.

   _____ Class I lesion   A. Incisal angle of anterior tooth

   _____ Class II lesion   B. Smooth proximal surfaces of anterior tooth

   _____ Class III lesion   C. Gingival third of lingual or facial surfaces

   _____ Class IV lesion   D. Proximal surfaces of posterior tooth

   _____ Class V lesion   E. Pit or fissure of an anterior tooth

10. Which of the following terms identifies an anatomic curvature of the occlusal alignment of the teeth, beginning at the cusp tip of the mandibular canine, following the buccal cusps of the premolars and molars, and continuing to the anterior border of the ramus?
    A. Curve of Spee
    B. Leeway space
    C. Primate spacing
    D. Centric occlusion

Learning Activities

1. Explain the purpose of pulp testing and how this procedure is performed.

_____

_____

_____

_____

_____

_____

_____

2. Describe how to calculate overjet and overbite. _____

_____

_____

_____

_____

_____

_____

_____

3. Report on a new technology for use in the identification of caries. _____

_____

_____

_____

_____

_____

_____

Board Style Review Questions

1. The chipping or flaking of enamel on the facial surface at the cervical third of the tooth is referred to as:
   A. Abfraction
   B. Abrasion
   C. Attrition
   D. Erosion
   E. Hypocalcification

2. White spots or a pitted appearance on the enamel surface is:
   A. Decalcification
   B. Erosion
   C. Hypocalcification
   D. Hypoplasia

3. Class II occlusion with division I occurs when one or more maxillary anterior teeth are inclined laterally and a lateral incisor is positioned labially. Division II occurs when one or more maxillary anterior teeth protrude facially.
   A. Both statements are true.
   B. The first statement is true; the second statement is false.
   C. Both statements are false.
   D. The first statement is false; the second statement is true.

4. In Angle's classification for occlusion, class III is described as:
   A. The mesiobuccal cusp of the maxillary first molar lies distal to the buccal groove of the mandibular first molar.
   B. The mesiobuccal cusp of the maxillary first permanent molar is positioned in the mesiobuccal groove of the mandibular first molar.
   C. The mesiobuccal cusp of the maxillary first molar lies mesial to the buccal groove of the mandibular first molar.

5. Vertical overlap of the maxillary anterior teeth with the mandibular teeth is called:
   A. Edge-to-edge bite
   B. End-to-end bite
   C. Open bite
   D. Overbite
   E. Underjet

6. Select the term that describes a situation in which the incisal surfaces of maxillary teeth occlude with the incisal edges of the mandibular teeth instead of overlapping.
   A. Edge-to-edge bite
   B. End-to-end bite
   C. Open bite
   D. Overbite
   E. Underjet

7. Select all of the statements that correctly describe the Universal Numbering System.
   1) It starts with the maxillary left third molar and ends with the maxillary right molar.
   2) It starts with the mandibular right third molar and ends with the mandibular left third molar.
   3) It starts with the maxillary right third molar and ends with the maxillary left molar.
   4) It starts with the mandibular left third molar and ends with the mandibular right third molar.
      A. 1 and 2
      B. 1 and 3
      C. 2 and 3
      D. 2 and 4
      E. 3 and 4

8. Identify the statement that describes centric occlusion.
   A. Spacing that is preserved during the mixed dentition period to allow for adequate space for the permanent dentition to erupt.
   B. Spacing in the primary dentition between the maxillary lateral and canine, and mandibular canine and first molar.
   C. The voluntary position of the dentition that allows the maximum contact when the teeth occlude.
   D. The anatomic curvature of the occlusal alignment of the teeth

9. Which of the following describes an end-to-end bite?
   A. Maxillary or mandibular posterior teeth are positioned either facial or lingual to their normal position.
   B. The incisal surfaces of maxillary teeth occlude with the incisal edges of mandibular teeth instead of overlapping.
   C. Molars and premolars occlude cusp to cusp.
   D. Lack of occlusal or incisal contact between the maxillary and mandibular teeth. The teeth do not occlude.

10. How would tooth #14 be identified in the International Standards Organization Designation System (ISO System)?
    A. 1 to 6
    B. 2 to 6
    C. 1 to 14
    D. 2 to 14
    E. 14

11. Class I occlusion with a tendency toward a class III is defined as:
    A. The mesial cusp of the maxillary first molar is mesial to the central groove of the mandibular molar by less than the width of a premolar.
    B. The mesiobuccal cusp of the maxillary first permanent molar is positioned in the mesiobuccal groove of the mandibular first molar.
    C. The mesial cusp of the maxillary first molar is distal to the central groove of the mandibular molar by less than the width of a premolar.

Active Learning

Refer to the photograph and Table 12-1 to respond to the following questions.

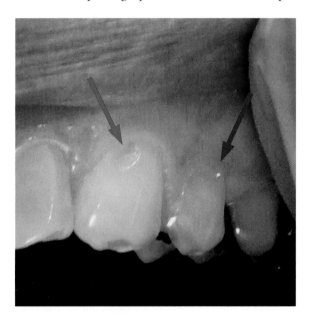

Procedure/ Condition	Pencil Color	Write in Tooth Box Above Tooth	Graphic/Drawing on Dental Chart
Amalgam	Blue		Outline restoration as accurately as possible and color in solid blue.
Anterior crowding	Lead pencil		Draw an arc from canine to canine on the lingual view and mark "ant cr" on the arc line.
Caries/decay	Red		Outline lesion and color in solid red.
Crown–porcelain/metal	Blue	PGVC (porcelain gold veneer crown) PM (porcelain to metal crown)	Outline ceramic crown in blue. Color metal portion solid blue. Write the type of crown in the tooth box above the tooth.
Defective restoration or poor margin integrity	Red		Outline the restoration in red.
Diastema	Lead pencil		Draw parallel lines at the location of the diastema on all views of the dental chart.

Table 12-1. **Dental Charting Symbols**

Continued

Table 12-1. *Dental Charting Symbols—cont'd*

Procedure/ Condition	Pencil Color	Write in Tooth Box Above Tooth	Graphic/Drawing on Dental Chart
Edentulous arch	Lead pencil		Draw an "X" from the upper-most aspect of one-third molar (#1) to the lowermost aspect of the third molar on the opposite side (#16). Indicate a denture by placing a check mark in the appliance box.
Fixed partial denture (bridge–pontic, abutment)	Lead pencil	PGVC, PM, gold crown (GC), etc	Draw a horizontal line immediately above or below the crowns of the bridge on the lingual view. Place a check mark in the appliance box.
Fixed retainer	Blue	NM (nonmetallic)	Draw the retainer on the lingual view as seen in the mouth. If applicable, chart any NM material and print NM in the tooth box.
Food impaction	Red		Draw an arrow on the lingual view of the chart to show interproximal areas of food impaction.
Fractured tooth	Red	RT (if root tip is retained)	Draw a zigzag line on the tooth where the fracture occurred. Place an "X" over the entire crown if it entirely fractured and RT is retained.
GC, gold foil (GF), gold inlay(GI), onlay	Blue	GC, GF, GI	Outline crown or restoration and draw diagonal lines.
Implant	Red	I	"X" out root in lead pencil notate bridgework/crown as usual.
Incipient caries	Red		Outline areas in red.
Malposed tooth 1. Drifting	Lead pencil		Place arrow in box indicating the direction the tooth has drifted.
Malposed tooth 2. Torsoversion	Lead pencil		Draw a curved arrow in the tooth box to indicate the proper direction the tooth is rotated.
Malposed tooth 3. Linguoversion, buccoversion, or labioversion	Lead pencil		Draw straight arrows in the tooth box to indicate the direction the tooth has moved.
Malposed tooth 4. Supraerupted or infraversion	Lead pencil		Place arrows on the lingual view of the tooth showing the direction of supraversion or infraversion.

Table 12-1. *Dental Charting Symbols—cont'd*

Procedure/ Condition	Pencil Color	Write in Tooth Box Above Tooth	Graphic/Drawing on Dental Chart
Maryland bridge, cantilever and fixed bridge	Blue	PGVC, PM, porcelain crown (PC)	Draw a horizontal line immediately above or below the crown of the bridge on the lingual view.
Missing tooth	Lead pencil		If the tooth has been replaced by a fixed prosthesis, "X" out the root only. Draw an "X" through the root and crown if the root has been replaced by a removable prosthesis.
Mixed dentition	Lead pencil	PE (partially erupted) UE (unerupted)	Draw an "X" through all missing deciduous teeth on the deciduous tooth chart. Write PE or UE in the tooth box of the permanent dentition.
NM restoration	Blue	NM (nonmetallic) PC	Outline the restoration as accurately as possible. Write NM or PC in the tooth box.
Recession	Blue		Measure the amount of recession from the CEJ and draw a blue line indicating recession on the tooth root.
Removable partial denture	Lead pencil		Place a check mark in the appliance box.
Retained deciduous tooth	Lead pencil	Print the letter of the deciduous tooth	"X" out the missing permanent tooth.
Root canal therapy	Blue	RC	Draw a line through the root canal on both the facial and lingual views.
Sealant (S)	Blue	S	Outline sealed areas in blue.
Supernumerary tooth	Blue		Draw on chart as close to their anatomic location and size as possible.
Temporary crown (TC)	Blue	TC	If temporary is metal.
Temporary restoration (T)	Blue	T	Outline in blue pencil.
Unerupted or partially erupted tooth	Lead pencil	UE, PE	
Veneer (V)	Blue	V	Outline restoration in blue if nonmetallic and color in solid.

Your patient is a 40-year-old female who presents with no pertinent medical concerns and takes no medications. After review of her history, you note that she consumes a low-carbohydrate diet and self-reports a history of bruxism. The patient reports no dental pain or sensitivity and states, "I just need my teeth cleaned."

1. Identify the shiny, noncarious lesion depicted by the blue arrow.
   A. Abfraction
   B. Abrasion
   C. Attrition
   D. Erosion

2. Identify the noncarious lesion depicted by the red arrow.
   A. Abfraction
   B. Abrasion
   C. Attrition
   D. Erosion

3 For dental charting, how should the clinician document the restoration on tooth #12?
   A. Outline and color in with a lead pencil
   B. Outline with red
   C. Outline with blue
   D. Outline and color in solid blue

4. Which of these is most important for the dental hygienist to discuss with the patient?
   A. At-home fluoride rinses
   B. Night guard
   C. Nutrition
   D. Tooth brushing technique

Rubrics/Process Evaluations

Process Evaluation Template		
Hard Tissue Examination		
Evaluation Criteria	**Criteria Met? (Y/N)**	**Comments**
Student records any missing, rotated, fractured, or unerupted teeth.		
Student charts any existing restorations.		
Student differentiates between types of restoration.		
Student records any endodontic restorations present.		
Student documents carious lesions.		
Student records any planned restorative procedures.		
Student properly records fixed bridge restorations.		
Student identifies and records implants.		
Full and/or partial dentures are noted.		
Presence of abfraction, attrition, abrasion, and/or erosion recorded.		
Presence of hypocalcification, hypoplasia, and/or decalcification recorded.		
Evidence of critical thinking/decision-making by student after review of histories (physician referral, consultation, determination of premedication requirements, etc.)		
Student conducted a thorough patient interview using appropriate probing questions to elicit accurate information.		
Patient interview conducted in an appropriate setting. Patient seated upright and at eye level to student.		

Chapter 13 | Biofilm, Calculus, and Stain

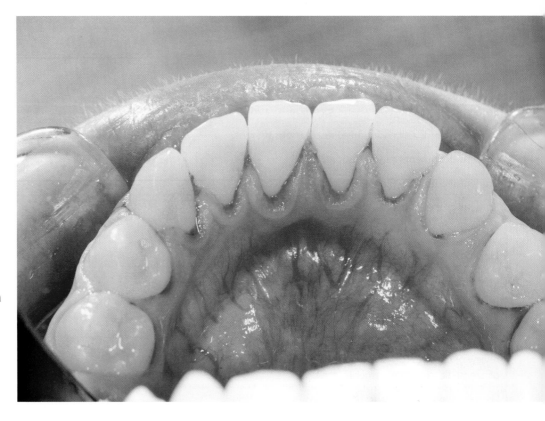

LEARNING OBJECTIVES

After reading this chapter, the student should be able to:

13.1 Define *biofilm* and *calculus*.

13.2 Identify the types of intrinsic and extrinsic stains.

13.3 Recognize the key microbes contained in bacterial biofilm.

13.4 List the different types of extrinsic stains and their cause.

13.5 Discuss the effects bacterial biofilm has on the oral cavity.

13.6 Give examples of different ways to detect calculus.

KEY CONCEPTS

- Reduction in biofilm growth will decrease the risk of periodontal disease and caries development.
- Accurate calculus detection and removal are important measures for an individual's overall health.
- The inflammatory process links periodontal disease to other chronic illnesses.

RELEVANCE TO CLINICAL PRACTICE

There are two types of deposits in the oral cavity: soft deposits (biofilm, pellicle, material alba, and food debris) and hard deposits (**calculus**). All deposits can attach to teeth, soft tissue, prosthetics, and restorative materials. The dental hygienist should identify soft and hard deposits, upon careful initial assessment of the patient's intraoral cavity.

Poor or neglected oral hygiene and diet are the two most common risk factors for caries formation. The regular removal of dental plaque biofilm, which contains the bacteria responsible for caries formation, gingivitis, and periodontitis, is the basis for maintaining dental health.[1] Mechanical disruption of the community structure of biofilm is necessary before damaging effects develop on the soft and hard tissue. Methods to control caries formation and periodontitis should include the prevention of biofilm growth.

The Basics

1 A reduction in which of the following will decrease the risk of periodontal disease?
   A. Acquired pellicle
   B. Biofilm
   C. Calcium and phosphate salts
   D. Calculus

2. Calculus can attach to:
   1) Prosthetics
   2) Restorative materials
   3) Soft tissue
      A. 1 and 2
      B. 2 and 3
      C. 1, 2, and 3
      D. Only 3

3. A thin film that coats the tooth immediately upon exposure to saliva is:
   A. Acquired pellicle
   B. Biofilm
   C. Calculus
   D. Materia alba

4. Which of these bacteria prefer a higher oxygen level?
   A. *Actinomyces*
   B. *Capnocytophaga*
   C. *Fusobacteria*
   D. *Streptococcus*

5. Select the type of soft deposit that defines reversible–irreversible attachment of the colonizing bacteria on the tooth surface.
   A. Biofilm
   B. Calculus
   C. Materia Alba
   D. Pellicle formation

6. A naturally occurring soft, sticky deposit in the oral cavity is:
   A. Biofilm
   B. Calculus
   C. Materia alba
   D. Pellicle formation

7. Calculus mineralization occurs in:
   A. 0 to 12 hours
   B. 24 to 72 hours
   C. 3 days
   D. 12 days

8. What gives subgingival calculus a dark to black color?

   _____

   _____

   _____

   _____

   _____

   _____

   _____

   _____

9. Distinguish between materia alba and dental biofilm.

   _____

   _____

   _____

   _____

   _____

   _____

   _____

   _____

10. Describe the three forms of calculus.

   1) _____

   _____

   _____

   _____

   2) _____

   _____

   _____

   _____

   3) _____

   _____

   _____

   _____

Learning Activities

1. Discuss the factors that can contribute to halitosis.

_____

_____

_____

_____

_____

_____

_____

2. Define the term *glycocalyx.*

_____

_____

_____

_____

_____

_____

_____

Board Style Review Questions

1. All of the following are correct descriptors of acquired pellicle *except* for one. Which one is the *exception?*
   A. Can be removed with tooth brushing
   B. Is a nonmineralized deposit
   C. Protects the tooth from acids that can cause demineralization of the enamel surface
   D. Thin film that coats the tooth immediately upon exposure to saliva

2. Which type of explorer can be used for calculus detection in a normal sulci or shallow pocket?
   1) 11/12 explorer
   2) Curved explorer
   3) Pigtail explorer
      A. 1 and 2
      B. 1 and 3
      C. 2 and 3
      D. 1, 2, and 3

3. Intrinsic endogenous stain can be caused by:
   A. Chlorhexidine 0.12% Rinses
   B. Coffee
   C. Tetracycline
   D. Tobacco

4. Black-line stain is caused by:
   A. Cigarettes, cigars, pipes, and tobacco chew
   B. Microorganisms that are mineralized on the tooth surface
   C. Microorganisms in an intermicrobial substance
   D. Chemical alteration of pellicle

5. Yellow stain is caused by:
   A. Cigarettes, cigars, pipes, and tobacco chew
   B. Microorganisms that are mineralized on the tooth surface
   C. Microorganisms in an intermicrobial substance
   D. Chemical alteration of pellicle

6. All of the following are descriptors of supragingival calculus *except* for one. Which one is the *exception?*
   A. Salivary calculus
   B. Located above the gingival margin
   C. Forms apical to the gingival margin
   D. Can form layers that encircle the tooth

7. Select the extrinsic stain that is usually seen on the cervical third of the tooth.
   A. Black-line
   B. Brown
   C. Orange
   D. Yellow

8. Choose the characteristics of mature biofilm.
   1) Gram-negative
   2) Gram-positive
   3) Aerobic
   4) Anaerobic
      A. 1 and 3
      B. 1 and 4
      C. 2 and 3
      D. 2 and 4

9. All of the following bacteria are associated with acquired pellicle and biofilm *except* for one. Which one is the *exception?*
   A. *Actinomyces viscosis*
   B. *Actinomycetemcomitans*
   C. *Streptococcus mutans*
   D. *Streptococcus sanguinis*

Critical Thinking/Clinical Reasoning Case Study

Refer to the photo to answer the following questions.

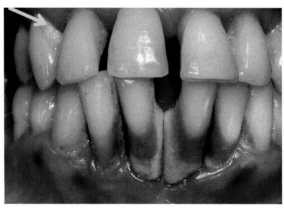

Photo courtesy of Phillip Dunn, DDS

1. Identify the type of stain in the photo covering the supragingival calculus along the mandibular central incisors.
   A. Intrinsic endogenous stain
   B. Intrinsic exogenous stain
   C. Extrinsic stain
   D. Tetracycline stain

2. Name the thick white cottage cheese-like deposit depicted by the yellow arrow.
   A. Acquired pellicle
   B. Biofilm
   C. Food debris
   D. Materia alba

3. The formation of calculus seen on the mandibular central incisors is best described as:
   A. Calculus ledges
   B. Calculus nodules
   C. Calculus rings
   D. Calculus spicules

REFERENCE

1. Gorur A, Lyle D, Schaudinn C. Biofilm removal with a dental waterjet. *Compend Contin Educ Dent.* 2009;30(Spec No 1):1-6.

Chapter 14 | Indices

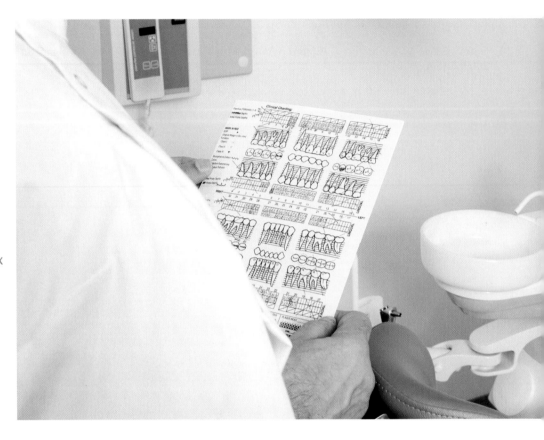

LEARNING OBJECTIVES

After reading this chapter, the student should be able to:

14.1 Describe the characteristics of a suitable or ideal index.

14.2 Explain the advantages and disadvantages of a useful index and indicate if it is appropriate for monitoring dental hygiene patients.

14.3 Choose a periodontal assessment tool for a new patient to determine: (a) periodontal problem, (b) treatment plan, (c) risk factors for future disease, (d) patient education plan, and (e) sequence of appointments.

14.4 Explain how indices are useful as an epidemiological tool.

14.5 Discuss the relationship of indices to evidence-based practice.

KEY CONCEPTS

• Oral indices translate a clinical picture into a numerical tool for comparisons of interest to characterize oral health status and provide evidence-based dental and dental hygiene care.

• Oral indices are helpful tools in risk assessment and needs assessment.

• Selection of an index depends on the question of interest or the purpose of evaluation.

• Indices provide feedback that determines success of care or opportunities for modifying patient care.

RELEVANCE TO CLINICAL PRACTICE

Assessment of the oral condition of the dental patient is essential to determine his or her current status of health and cleanliness, and it serves as the basis for problem identification or diagnoses and therapeutic interventions (see Application to Clinical Practice 1). One of the tools for oral health assessment is a clinical **index**, which is simply a scoring system or measuring device. For example, the periodontal probe can be used like a ruler to measure the height of calculus on the six mandibular lingual incisor teeth (Volpe-Manhold Index [VMI]) or to measure the depth of the gingival sulcus (clinical probing depth). An index used for oral health assessment can be a tool for evaluating, educating, and motivating the patient; it can be used to create a treatment plan and to monitor changes over time to measure the success of personal disease-control efforts. Indices can be used to help a patient recognize an oral problem, reveal the proficiency of current oral hygiene procedures, motivate a patient to eliminate or control oral disease, and evaluate the success of patient and professional treatment over a period. Indices are also an important tool for documentation and recordkeeping. Indices may also provide some measure of the dental hygienist's capability, not only as an educator or motivator but also as a clinician. Indices can be a reflection of the success of types of services provided.

The Basics

1. The Ramfjord teeth include:
   A. #3, 8, 12, 19, 24, 28
   B. #3, 9, 14, 19, 25, 30
   C. #3, 9, 12, 19, 25, 28
   D. #2, 8, 13, 18, 24, 30

2. Analysis of data collected from 2009 to 2010 by the National Institute for Dental Research (NIDR) indicated that the prevalence of periodontitis was far higher than in previous epidemiological surveys. What contributed to the underestimation of the true prevalence of periodontitis?

_____

_____

_____

_____

_____

_____

_____

_____

_____

_____

3. This index is generally used for research purposes to evaluate tartar-control products.
   A. Simplified calculus index
   B. Russell periodontal index
   C. Periodontal index
   D. Volpe-Manhold Index

4. Select the oral hygiene index that is commonly used to measure plaque removal effectiveness of different toothbrush designs.
   A. Plaque control record
   B. Rustogi modification of the Navy Plaque Index
   C. Silness Löe Plaque Index
   D. Turesky modification of the Quigley-Hein Plaque Index

5. Select the gingival health index that is noninvasive and strictly visual.
   A. Eastman Interdental Bleeding Index
   B. Modified gingival index
   C. Gingival bleeding index
   D. Periodontal disease index

6. All of the following indices use disclosing solution to identify plaque biofilm *except* for one. Which one is the *exception?*
   A. Plaque Control Record
   B. Rustogi modification of the Navy Plaque Index
   C. Silness Löe Plaque Index
   D. Turesky modification of the Quigley-Hein Plaque Index

7. All of the following are true of the Oral Hygiene Index (OHI) *except* for one. Which one is the *exception?*
   A. Allows for the patient's oral cleanliness to be assessed from visit to visit.
   B. All teeth present are scored.
   C. Surfaces covered with plaque/debris are evaluated.
   D. The tip of a probe or explorer is used.

8. Which index can be used to identify individuals with the highest caries values in a particular population?
   A. Significant caries index (SiC)
   B. Volpe-Manhold Index
   C. Caries-Risk Assessment Tool (CAT)
   D. Caries Management by Risk Assessment (CAMBRA)

9. For the decayed, missing, filled teeth (DMFT) index, what score is assigned to a missing tooth for any other reason than decay?
   A. 3
   B. 4
   C. 5
   D. 6

10. For the DMFT index, a score of 9 represents:
    A. Erupted teeth that can not be examined
    B. Trauma
    C. Teeth with sealants
    D. A missing tooth as a result of decay

Learning Activities

1. Explain the characteristics of an ideal index.

_____

_____

_____

_____

_____

_____

_____

_____

_____

2. Compare and contrast computer-generated risk assessment models such as PreViser, Oral Health Information Suite (OHIS), and the Periodontal Risk Calculator (PRC).

_____

_____

_____

_____

_____

_____

_____

_____

_____

_____

Board Style Review Questions

1. Select the best definition for the term *prevalence*.
   A. A means of assessing oral hygiene status by measuring criteria.
   B. Extent to which new cases exist within a population.
   C. A method of converting the observed severity of a parameter of interest into a numerical form.
   D. The total number of people manifesting a particular condition.

2. All of the following indices measure oral hygiene status *except* for one. Which one is the *exception?*
   A. Oral Hygiene Index
   B. Periodontal scoring and recording index
   C. Plaque control record
   D. Rustogi modification of the Navy Plaque Index

3. The DMFT is an index that represents:
   A. Decayed, missing, and filled primary teeth
   B. Decayed, missing, and filled surfaces of primary teeth
   C. Decayed, missing, and filled permanent teeth
   D. Decayed, missing, and filled surfaces of permanent teeth

4. Select the bleeding index that uses a wooden pick to assess.
   A. Eastman Interdental Bleeding Index
   B. Gingival bleeding index
   C. Modified gingival index
   D. Volpe-Manhold Index

5. Identify the level of measurement that has distinct definitions for each score in a graduated scale.
   A. Dichotomous scale
   B. Nominal scale
   C. Ordinal scale
   D. Reversible scale

6. The presence or absence of bleeding is considered a(an):
   A. Dichotomous scale
   B. Interval scale
   C. Ordinal scale
   D. Ratio scale

7. Choose the bleeding index that uses floss to elicit bleeding.
   A. Eastman Interdental Bleeding Index
   B. Gingival bleeding index
   C. Modified gingival index
   D. Gingival index

8. Select the term that best identifies between-examiner agreement.
   A. Intraexaminer reliability
   B. Interexaminer reliability
   C. Dichotomous
   D. Reversible indices

9. Choose any of the following that describe the Russell periodontal index:
   1) Measures clinical attachment levels (CAL)
   2) Measures the condition of the gingiva and bone individually
   3) Provides overall periodontal disease prevalence in a large population
      A. 1 and 2
      B. 1 and 3
      C. 2 and 3
      D. Only 3

10. Which periodontal health status index evaluates bleeding, deposits, and pocket depth?
    A. Russell periodontal index
    B. Periodontal disease index
    C. Periodontal screening Examination
    D. Volpe-Manhold Index

Active Learning

Refer to this photo to answer the following questions.

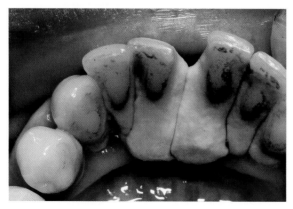

Photo courtesy of Phillip Dunn, DDS

1. Identify the most appropriate indices for measuring the calculus seen in this photo.
   A. Ramfjord teeth index
   B. Russell periodontal index
   C. Taresky modification of the Quigley-Hein Plaque Index
   D. Volpe-Manhold Index

2. The indices in question 1 can be used as an oral health assessment tool. Which of the following is not a function of this index?
    A. To educate and motivate the patient
    B. To create a treatment plan
    C. To assess the prevalence of the dental disease
    D. To help the patient recognize an oral problem

3. Based on the simplified calculus index, the calculus in the photo would be given a score of:
    A. 1
    B. 2
    C. 3
    D. 4

Chapter 15 | Radiology

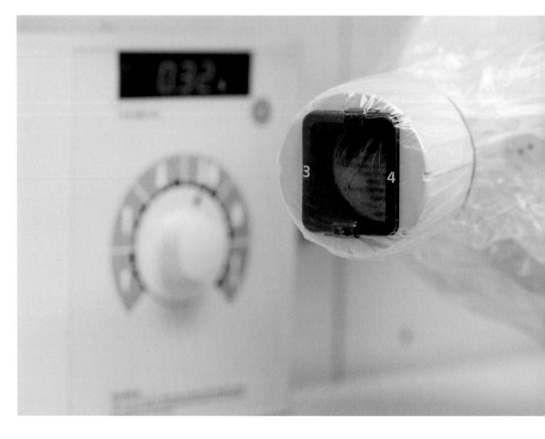

LEARNING OBJECTIVES

After reading this chapter, the student should be able to:

15.1 Describe properties of x-rays.

15.2 Describe and correctly use basic radiology terms when working with other dental professionals and patients.

15.3 Identify normal radiographic appearances of teeth and surrounding structures on radiographs.

15.4 Describe analog film versus digital imaging systems.

15.5 Describe ionizing radiation protection guidelines.

KEY CONCEPTS

• Basic radiographic terms are important when working with other dental professionals.

• Knowledge of the different types of imaging systems in dentistry is beneficial when working in a dental office.

• Responsible use of ionizing radiation is necessary to ensure patients are exposed to the least amount of radiation possible.

RELEVANCE TO CLINICAL PRACTICE

Radiographs show information including, but not limited to, location and quantity of calculus, bone defects, furcation involvement, and restorative margin defects. This information allows the dental hygienist to formulate optimum treatment plans for patients to aid in their efforts to improve or maintain their at-home oral health care.

The Basics

1. The type of intraoral radiograph that is most commonly used to evaluate the bone around the apex of a tooth is a(an):
   A. Bitewing
   B. Occlusal
   C. Panoramic
   D. Periapical

2. Which component of analog film is used to prevent backscatter radiation from decreasing image quality?
   A. Base emulsion
   B. Black paper
   C. Lead foil
   D. Adhesive layer

3. What is the total average radiation dose attributed to radiation exposure in dentistry?
   A. 5% to 7%
   B. 3% to 5%
   C. 1% to 3%
   D. Less than 1%

4. Which of the following phrases relate to stochastic effects?
   1) Radiation dose and response severity are proportional
   2) All-or-nothing effects
   3) Radiation-induced damage will or will not occur
   4) Dose-dependent effects
      A. 1 and 2
      B. 1 and 4
      C. 2 and 3
      D. 3 and 4

5. The average background radiation dose a person is exposed to in 1 year ranges from:
   A. 120 mSv to 160 mSv
   B. 360 mSv to 620 mSv
   C. 760 mSv to 820 mSv
   D. 660 mSv to 1000 mSv

6. If the dental hygienist uses a rectangular collimation with the same settings as a round collimation, the resulting radiation exposure to the patient will be:
   A. Decreased
   B. Increased
   C. Stays the same

7. All of the following are types of extraoral radiographs *except* for one. Which one is the *exception?*
   A. Lateral cephalometric skull radiograph
   B. Occlusal radiograph
   C. Orthopantomograph
   D. Panoramic

8. Refer to the guidelines for prescribing dental radiographs from the ADA and the FDA. What is the suggested time frame for exposing a posterior bitewing examination on an adolescent recall patient with no clinical caries and not at increased risk for caries?
   A. 6 to 18 months
   B. 12 to 24 months
   C. 18 to 36 months
   D. 24 to 36 months

9. Size 1 film is commonly used for:
   1) Periapicals on children
   2) Bitewings on children
   3) Posterior periapicals on adults
   4) Anterior periapicals on adults
      A. 1 and 2
      B. 1, 2, and 3
      C. 1, 2, and 4
      D. Only 2

10. Define collimation.
    A. Background radiation
    B. Absorption and storage of energy when exposed by x-rays
    C. Dose equivalence
    D. Shaping the x-ray beam to the area that is to be imaged

Learning Activities

1. Describe the precautions an operator should take to ensure that he/she is exposed to a minimal amount of ionizing radiation.

_____

_____

_____

_____

_____

_____

_____

_____

_____

_____

_____

_____

_____

_____

_____

_____

2. Compare and contrast analog film versus digital imaging.

_____

_____

_____

_____

_____

_____

_____

_____

_____

_____

_____

_____

_____

_____

_____

_____

_____

Board Style Review Questions

1. Dentin and enamel appear radiopaque on radiographs. The pulp chamber and root canal appear radiolucent.
   A. Both statements are correct.
   B. The first statement is correct; the second statement is incorrect.
   C. Both statements are incorrect.
   D. The first statement is incorrect; the second statement is correct.

2. Choose the best description for a latent image.
   A. Created only on digital imaging.
   B. Created only on an analog x-ray film.
   C. An image that is not visible to the naked eye until it is processed.
   D. An image that is visible to the naked eye.

3. Select the type of radiograph that is ideal for evaluating bone levels.
   A. Bitewing
   B. Occlusal
   C. Panorex
   D. Periapical

4. Identify the term(s) that refer to the amount of black, white, and gray on a final radiograph.
   1) Contrast
   2) Density
   3) Radiolucent
   4) Radiopaque
      A. Only 1
      B. 1 and 2
      C. 1 and 3
      D. 3 and 4

5. A radiograph with high contrast will show changes in grays and have less black and white areas on the image. A radiograph with low contrast will be an overall gray image with little change in the grays throughout the image.
   A. Both statements are true.
   B. The first statement is true; the second statement is false.
   C. Both statements are false.
   D. The first statement is false; the second statement is true.

6. The smaller the grain size, the shorter the exposure time for analog film. Therefore, because of its grain size, the F speed film requires the least radiation exposure to the patient.
   A. Both the statement and the reason are correct.
   B. The statement is correct; the reason is incorrect.
   C. Both the statement and the reason are incorrect.
   D. The statement is incorrect; the reason is correct.

7. Pick the term that labels the principle of maximizing diagnostic yield while minimizing patient exposure.
   A. Computed radiography
   B. Justification
   C. Optimization
   D. Stochastic effect

8. A radiograph can be defined as:
   A. Production of ions as they travel through matter.
   B. Maximized diagnostic yield.
   C. The resultant image after a patient is exposed to x-rays.
   D. An image that is not visible to the naked eye.

9. The term radiolucent refers to:
   1) Areas that block the transmission of x-rays
   2) Areas that appear light or white
   3) X-rays that are transmitted to the image receptor
   4) Areas that appear dark or black
      A. 1 and 2
      B. 1 and 4
      C. 2 and 3
      D. 3 and 4

10. Choose the type of radiograph used frequently in orthodontics to evaluate the position of the jaws in relation to each other and the skull base.
    A. Lateral cephalometric skull radiograph
    B. Orthopantomograph
    C. Panoramic radiograph
    D. Pantomograph

Active Learning

Your patient is a 25-year-old female who has never been to the dentist. Use the radiograph provided to answer the following questions.

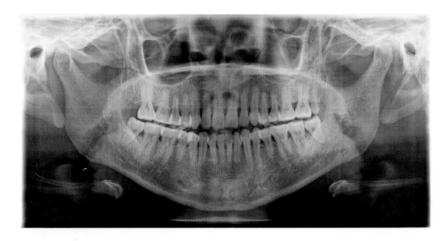

L

1. Identify the radiopacity associated with tooth #32.
   A. Periodontal ligament
   B. Dentin
   C. Calculus
   D. Lesion at the apex

2. Which of the following best describes this radiograph?
   A. Ideal contrast
   B. High contrast
   C. Low contrast
   D. High density
   E. Low density

3. The radiolucency surrounding tooth #31 is:
   A. Calculus
   B. Dentin
   C. Enamel
   D. Periodontal ligament

Chapter 16 | Dietary Assessment and Nutritional Counseling

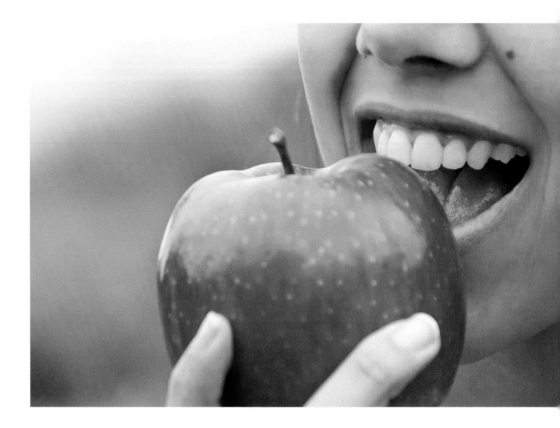

LEARNING OBJECTIVES

After reading this chapter, the student should be able to:

16.1 Recognize dietary factors that may increase a patient's risk for oral/dental conditions.

16.2 Recognize oral manifestations associated with nutrient imbalance.

16.3 Identify oral conditions that increase a patient's risk for nutrient imbalance.

16.4 Recognize the tools used to assess a patient's diet.

16.5 Demonstrate appropriate nutritional counseling procedures and communication skills.

16.6 Educate the patient about how diet impacts oral health and how oral health impacts diet.

16.7 Assist the patient in assessing the adequacy of his/her diet and the dietary risk factors to oral/dental health.

16.8 Recognize conditions that require a referral to a registered dietitian, physician, or both.

KEY CONCEPTS

- Oral/dental health affects diet and nutritional status.
- Diet and nutritional status affects oral/dental health.
- Diet screening, nutrition education, and guidance are essential components of clinical dental care.
- Good communication skills are critical to effective nutritional counseling.

RELEVANCE TO CLINICAL PRACTICE

Nutritional status, diet, and oral health are closely interrelated. A healthy dentition promotes good chewing function, and normal mastication is needed to support a healthy diet. Likewise, a healthy diet is needed to support and maintain optimal health of oral tissues. These relationships, along with the frequency of preventative dental care appointments, place the dental hygienist in an ideal position to screen patients for nutritional and oral health risk.

Dietary assessment or screening is considered an integral part of health promotion and disease prevention in comprehensive patient care.[1,2] Although all patients can benefit from dietary assessment, nutrition intervention is especially important when the patient's oral/dental conditions compromise dietary intake or the patient's diet represents an increased risk for oral/dental disease(s), or both.

The Basics

1. Complete the following table using Table 16-4 Estimated Calorie Needs Per Day By Age, Gender, and Physical Activity Level (Detailed) in your textbook as a reference.

Your patient is a...	Estimated Caloric Needs
25-year-old, moderately active male	
60-year-old, sedentary female	
10-year-old boy involved in basketball and football	
16-year-old female who walks to school every day and plays soccer	

2. Optimal salivary flow reduces the risk of dental disease by all of the following mechanisms *except* for one. Which one is the *exception?*
   A. Antimicrobial activity
   B. Reduced clearance of food from the oral cavity
   C. Promotes remineralization
   D. Buffers acids

3. List the nutrient deficiencies that can manifest in the following tissues.

Oral soft tissues   Hard tissues (teeth, bone)

a. _____   a. _____

b. _____   b. _____

c. _____   c. _____

d. _____   d. _____

e. _____   e. _____

                                               f. _____

4. Examine the sample 24 Hour Recall provided in Table 16-2 in your textbook. Identify the foods consumed during dinner that *do not* decrease plaque pH.

A. _____

_____

_____

B. _____

_____

_____

C. _____

_____

_____

5. Compare and contrast the Food Record and the 24 Hour Recall. Are both of these tools appropriate for screening the adequacy of your patient's diet? Why or why not? Explain which one you would use to evaluate your patient's caries risk.

_____

_____

_____

_____

_____

_____

_____

_____

_____

_____

_____

_____

_____

_____

_____

_____

_____

_____

6. All of the following nutrient deficiencies could contribute to the oral manifestation in the photo *except* for one. Which one is the *exception*?

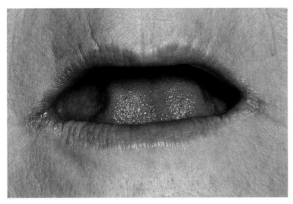

Photo courtesy of Carl Allen, DDS

    A. Vitamin D
    B. Niacin
    C. Iron
    D. Riboflavin
    E. Folate

7. How would you document informed consent for nutritional counseling? What would you include in your patient's record after nutritional counseling?

_____

_____

_____

_____

_____

_____

_____

_____

_____

_____

_____

_____

_____

Learning Activities

1. After your patient completes a food record, identify caries risk factors. Refer to Box 16-5 Dietary Guidelines to Reduce Dental Caries Risk in your textbook.

_____

_____

_____

_____

_____

2. Describe the role of the dental hygienist in dietary assessment as part of comprehensive patient care.

_____

_____

_____

_____

_____

_____

3. Identify conditions in which a referral to a dietitian/physician would be necessary.

_____

_____

_____

_____

_____

_____

4. Using the criteria provided in Table 16-1 Oral Signs Associated with Malnutrition in your textbook, role-play with a student partner to practice effective communication skills during a mock nutritional counseling session.

Board Style Review Questions

1. Refer to Table 16-1 Oral Signs Associated With Malnutrition in your textbook. From the following list, select all of the oral manifestations that may be associated with an iron deficiency.
   A. Angular chelitis
   B. Atrophic oral mucosa
   C. Beefy, red tongue
   D. Candidiasis
   E. Decreased alveolar bone integrity
   F. Glossitis
   G. Hypogeussa
   H. Mucositis

2. Order the steps in providing a dietary assessment to a patient. Match each letter with its proper sequence number.

Step 1 _____	a. Assess patient's progress
Step 2 _____	b. Provide nutrition education
Step 3 _____	c. Examine caloric needs
Step 4 _____	d. Document in patient record
Step 5 _____	e. Review the food record with the patient
Step 6 _____	f. Compare the actual amount consumed to the recommended amount for each food group
Step 7 _____	g. Review recommendations for food groups
Step 8 _____	h. Provide instructions to complete the food record
Step 9 _____	i. Examine the adequacy of his/her diet
Step 10 _____	j. Assist with dietary/lifestyle modifications
Step 11 _____	k. Review nutrition, exercise, dental, and health histories
Step 12 _____	l. Review dietary risk(s) for dental caries

3. Select the foods that decrease biofilm pH.
    1) Fruit juice
    2) Cucumber
    3) Pudding
    4) Cheese
    5) Rice
        A. 1, 2, 4
        B. 2, 4, 5
        C. 1, 3, 5
        D. 1 and 3 only

4. Understanding a patient's lifestyle and values can contribute to the success of long-term dietary changes; therefore, the dental hygienist should review the patient's dietary influences including cultural values and psychological factors.
    A. Both the statement and reason are correct and related.
    B. Both the statement and reason are correct but *not* related.
    C. The statement is correct, but the reason is *not*.
    D. The statement is *not* correct, but the reason is correct.
    E. *Neither* the statement *nor* the reason is correct.

5. Vitamins A and K are two of the water-soluble nutrients. Both vitamins A and K can be acquired from green leafy vegetables.
    A. Both statements are true.
    B. Both statements are false.
    C. The first statement is true; the second is false.
    D. The first statement is false; the second is true.

6. Your patient presents with a beefy red tongue. Which of the following vitamin deficiencies is *most* likely contributing to this condition?
    A. Vitamin A
    B. Vitamin B_3
    C. Vitamin B_{12}
    D. Vitamin C

7. During a risk assessment, all of the following are considerations for reducing dental caries risk *except* for one. Which one is the *exception*?
    A. The sequencing of food consumption.
    B. Identifying sources of dental erosion.
    C. Amount of fermentable carbohydrates in the diet.
    D. Utilization of xylitol-containing products.
    E. Determine appropriate water intake to reduce xerostomia.

8. Identify the role of the dental hygienist in nutritional counseling?
    1) Understanding the patient's readiness to change
    2) Instruct the patient to identify dietary and oral health risk on his/her own
    3) Provide nutrition and oral health education
    4) Promote positive change through behavior modification
        A. 1, 2, and 3
        B. 1, 3, and 4
        C. Only 1 and 4
        D. All of the above

9. Your patient has type 2 diabetes, is overweight, and has several areas of dental decay. After reviewing a 24 Hour Recall with this patient, you educate him on the cariogenic potential of a diet high in fermentable carbohydrates. What would be the *best* next step for this patient?
    A. Have the patient complete a food record for the next 3 days to get a more detailed overview of his dietary behaviors
    B. Review My Plate Guidelines
    C. Provide dietary modifications to improve health as related to diabetes
    D. Refer the patient to a registered dietitian and/or physician

Active Learning

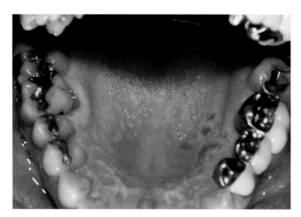

Photo courtesy of Phillip Dunn, DDS

This patient presented for dental hygiene care. He completed a 24 Hour Recall of his food and beverage consumption as follows. Breakfast: 2 scrambled eggs, 1 piece of white toast with butter, 1 cup of black coffee. Lunch: Small pepperoni pizza, 2 diet sodas. Snack: Potato chips, 1 diet soda. Dinner: Meatloaf, mashed potatoes and gravy, green beans, one 8-oz glass of milk. Breakfast: Cinnamon Roll, 1 cup of black coffee. Use this information and the photograph to answer the following questions.

1. Choose all that apply. Which nutrient imbalance(s) could be contributing to the condition seen in the photo?
    1) Vitamin B_1
    2) Vitamin B_{12}
    3) Folate
    4) Iron
        A. 1 and 2
        B. 1, 2, and 3
        C. 1, 2, 3, and 4
        D. Only 3

2. The primary purpose of a dietary assessment for this patient is to:
    A. Evaluate caries risk
    B. Reflect on day-to-day intake variability
    C. Emphasize nutritional needs
    D. Determine general dietary adequacy

3. List two recommendations that can be provided based on the 24 Hour Recall.

    1) _____

    _____

    _____

    2) _____

    _____

    _____

REFERENCES

1. Nappo-Dattoma L. Diet and dietary analysis. In: Koger B, ed. *Clinical Practice of the Dental Hygienist.* 10th ed. Philadelphia: Lippincott Williams & Wilkens; 2009:521-543.
2. Touger-Decker R, Sirois DA. Approaches to oral nutrition health risk assessment. In: Touger-Decker R, Sirois D, Mobley C, eds. *Nutrition and Oral Medicine.* Totowa, NJ: Humana Press; 2005:287-297.

Rubrics/Process Evaluations

Process Evaluation Template		
Nutrition Counseling		
Evaluation Criteria	**Criteria Met? (Y/N)**	**Comments**
Student provided rationale for patient selection.		
Procedure explained to patient and informed consent obtained and documented.		
Student provided instructions to the patient on completing the food record.		
Reviewed food record and patient histories.		
Student provided nutrition education.		
Caloric intake and food group amounts reviewed and compared with actual patient consumption.		
Reviewed dental caries risk assessment form and compared with dietary guidelines.		
Reviewed strategies with patient to improve diet/lifestyle.		
Nutritional counseling was documented in patient record.		
Student used standard precautions during procedure.		

Chapter 17 | Risk Assessment

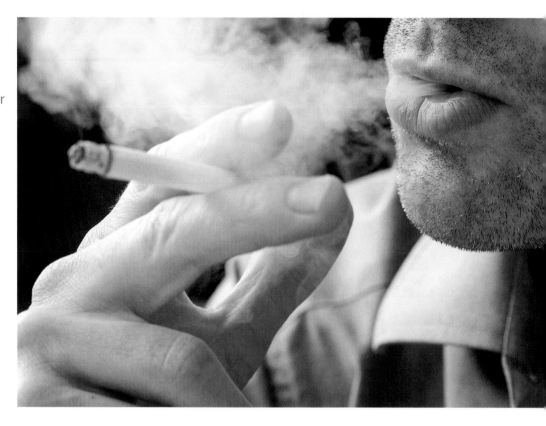

LEARNING OBJECTIVES

After reading this chapter, the student should be able to:

17.1 Discuss the relevance of risk assessment as part of dental hygiene practice.

17.2 Explain the difference among a risk factor, risk indicator, and risk marker.

17.3 Identify risk factors that affect the onset, severity, and progression of periodontal disease.

17.4 Differentiate between modifiable risk factors and nonmodifiable risk factors.

17.5 Explain the implications of a risk factor with a patient and implications for self-care regimen.

17.6 Discuss treatment recommendations for a patient who is genotype-positive.

17.7 Understand the difference between high-risk factors and low-risk factors.

17.8 Explain why diabetes, smoking, and genetics are significant risk factors.

17.9 Identify risk factors for oral cancer and dental caries.

17.10 Discuss the differences in risk for age, race, and genetics.

17.11 Develop a risk assessment form.

KEY CONCEPTS

- Risk assessment is the cornerstone to developing a patient-centered care plan.
- Risk factors modulate the onset, severity, and prognosis of periodontal diseases, dental caries, and oral cancer.
- The most significant periodontal risk factors are smoking, diabetes, and genetics.
- The most significant oral cancer risk factors are tobacco use, alcohol, and HPV.
- Reduction of risk factors improves therapy outcomes and prognosis.
- Patient compliance to self-care regimens and reduction of risk are important factors for the prevention or treatment of oral infectious diseases.

RELEVANCE TO CLINICAL PRACTICE

Preventing, eliminating, or managing oral inflammatory diseases depends on many factors: thorough documentation of clinical, historical, and biological data; patient behaviors and values; development of an individualized evidence-based care plan; and risk assessment. Risk assessment involves identifying patients who are at risk for developing oral disease such as periodontal disease, caries, and oral cancer. Assessing the patient's risk can have a significant impact on clinical decisions, interventions, and prognosis.[1–6]

Risk assessment, diagnosis, and presentation of a comprehensive care plan are the responsibility of the dentist and dental hygienist (see Professionalism). The patient's role is providing accurate and detailed information regarding medical and dental histories including personal habits and lifestyle behaviors, risk reduction by way of behavior change, incorporation of recommended self-care routine, and adherence to accepted care plan and continued care. This chapter discusses the impact of risk factors and the dental hygienist's role in patient assessment, education, and treatment planning.

The Basics

1. List three clinic components that are affected by assessing the patient's risk.

   1) _____

   2) _____

   3) _____

2. With regard to collection of patient demographic information, give an example of a risk indicator that is collected during the medical assessment of your patient.

_____

_____

_____

_____

_____

_____

_____

_____

3. What intraoral changes are often observed in patients using smokeless tobacco?

1) _____

2) _____

3) _____

4) _____

5) _____

4. Studies show that smokers have a _____ greater risk for periodontal disease than never smokers. _____ % of patients with oral cancer use tobacco. Oral cancer is _____ more frequent in alcoholic drinkers than nondrinkers.

5. Match the following risk assessment terms with the appropriate definition.

_____ Risk factor

_____ Risk marker

_____ Risk

_____ Risk assessment

_____ Risk indicator

A. Causal relationship not shown through research, associated relationship from population data, or data collected long-term

B. Evaluation of qualitative and quantitative data

C. Biologically plausible but only associated with disease through research

D. Probability that loss, harm, or injury will occur if nothing is changed

E. Behavior or attribute that has a direct causal effect on the onset and/or progression of the disease

6. List five clinical findings that can be observed in patients who smoke.

1) _____

2) _____

3) _____

4) _____

5) _____

7. Your patient presents with minimal biofilm, pale gingiva, and slight bleeding on probing. The assessments show generalized attachment loss with more significant periodontal destruction in the anterior regions. Explain how cellular and/or local effects of smoking could apply to this clinical condition.

_____

_____

_____

_____

_____

_____

_____

_____

_____

_____

_____

_____

8. Describe the effects of smoking on the following:

Wound healing: _____

_____

_____

_____

_____

Collagen production: _____

_____

_____

_____

_____

9. Explain why a patient with diabetes is at risk for periodontal disease and how periodontal disease influences the metabolism.

_____

_____

_____

_____

_____

_____

_____

_____

_____

Learning Activities

1. Explain the role of the dental hygienist in risk assessment.

_____

_____

_____

_____

_____

_____

_____

_____

2. Defend the belief that periodontal disease is more prevalent in older populations but not because it is an age-related risk factor.

_____

_____

_____

_____

_____

_____

_____

_____

3. Relate the genetic susceptibility test to periodontal disease.

_____

_____

_____

_____

_____

_____

_____

_____

4. Differentiate between genotype-positive and genotype-negative.

_____

_____

_____

_____

_____

_____

_____

5. Go to the American Academy of Periodontology website and practice using the risk assessment tool for periodontal disease.

Board Style Review Questions

1. Periodontal treatment outcomes are often based on the presence or absence of bleeding. For this reason, bleeding alone is a predictor of periodontal breakdown or future attachment loss.
   A. The statement and the reason are both correct.
   B. The statement is correct; the reason is incorrect.
   C. The statement and the reason are both incorrect.
   D. The statement is incorrect; the reason is correct.

2. The probability that a person will develop a disease after exposure to a risk factor compared with a person who has not been exposed to that same risk factor is termed:
   A. Odds ratio
   B. Relative risk
   C. Risk factor
   D. Prevalence

3. Identify the correct statement(s) as related to risk.
   1) Periodontal disease is more prevalent in older populations.
   2) Individuals from lower socioeconomic status have an increased risk for periodontal disease.
   3) Women have a higher prevalence for periodontal disease.
      A. 1 and 2
      B. Only 1
      C. 2 and 3
      D. All of the statements are correct

4. All of the following can result from xerostomia *except* for one. Which one is the *exception?*
   A. Difficulty chewing
   B. Burning mouth
   C. Mucositis
   D. Less acidic pH

5. Risk assessment is the responsibility of the dentist and dental hygienist. The patient's role in risk assessment is to provide accurate and detailed information regarding medical and dental histories.
   A. Both statements are true.
   B. The first statement is true; the second statement is false.
   C. Both statements are false.
   D. The first statement is false; the second statement is true.

6. Which of the following is a nonmodifiable risk factor?
   A. Age
   B. Tobacco use
   C. Faulty restorations
   D. Daily oral hygiene

7. Incidence is the total number of cases of a disease within the population at a specific point in time. Prevalence is the number of new cases of a disease over a specified period of time.
   A. Both statements are true.
   B. The first statement is true; the second is false.
   C. Both statements are false.
   D. The first statement is false; the second is true.

8. Select all of the following bacteria that are specific to caries.
   1) *Lactobacilli*
   2) *Porphyromonas gingivalis*
   3) *Aggregatibacter actinomycetemcomitans*
   4) *Mutans streptococci*
      A. 1, 2, and 3
      B. Only 1 and 4
      C. Only 3 and 4
      D. All of the above

9. Which of the following risk factors is the simplest to eliminate to help reduce periodontal disease risk?
   A. Age
   B. Genetics
   C. Inadequate oral hygiene
   D. Smoking

10. Smokers respond just as well to periodontal therapy as nonsmokers. A direct relationship exists between attachment loss and pack-years (number of years smoked).
   A. Both statements are correct
   B. The first statement is correct; the second is incorrect.
   C. Both statements are incorrect.
   D. The first statement is incorrect; the second statement is correct.

REFERENCES

1. Douglass CW. Risk assessment and management of periodontal disease. *J Am Dent Assoc.* 2006;137(suppl):27S-32S.
2. Page RC, Beck JD. Risk assessment for periodontal diseases. *Int Dent J.* 1997;47(2):61-87.
3. Beck JD. Methods of assessing risk for periodontitis and developing multifactorial models. *J Periodontol.* 1994;65(suppl 5):468-478.
4. Page R, Krall EA, Martin J, et al. Validity and accuracy of a risk calculator in predicting periodontal disease. *J Am Dent Assoc.* 2002;133(5):569-576.
5. Nunn ME. Understanding the etiology of periodontitis: an overview of periodontal risk factors. *Periodontol 2000.* 2003;32:11-23.
6. Pihlstrom BL. Periodontal risk assessment, diagnosis and treatment planning. *Periodontol 2000.* 2001;25:37-58.

Rubrics/Process Evaluations

Process Evaluation Template

Systematic Process for Risk Assessment

Evaluation Criteria	Criteria Met? (Y/N)	Comments
Assessment: Gather and review patient data.		
Analysis: Data analyzed for oral risk.		
Dental hygiene diagnosis: Identification of existing or potential oral health problems within the scope of practice of the dental hygienist.		
Plan: Identification of outcome goals, patient-centered interventions, and changes in modifiable risk factors.		
Implementation: Delivery of dental hygiene services and consultations.		
Evaluation: Evaluation of outcomes and adjustment of care plan as needed.		
Student uses standard precautions during procedure.		
Documentation in patient record.		

Part V

Diagnosis and Planning

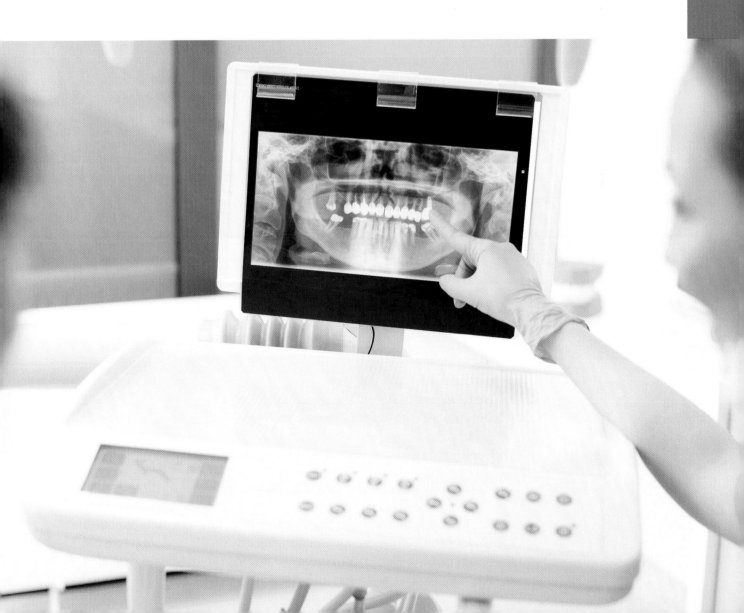

Chapter 18 | Dental Hygiene Diagnosis, Treatment Plan, Documentation, and Case Presentation

120

KEY TERMS

battery
breach of contract
definitive diagnosis
differential diagnosis
expressed consent
implied consent
informed consent
informed refusal
treatment plan

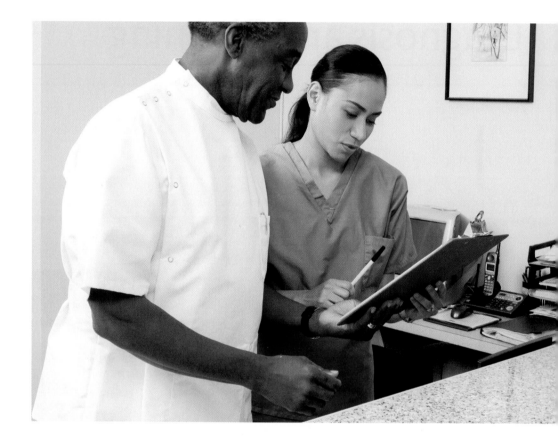

LEARNING OBJECTIVES

After reading this chapter, the student should be able to:

18.1 Analyze and interpret all assessment data to determine a differential diagnosis.

18.2 Use critical thinking skills to determine the definitive dental hygiene diagnosis.

18.3 Develop a dental hygiene treatment plan.

18.4 Develop a case presentation for the patient, caregiver, dentist, or other health-care providers.

18.5 Document the case consistent with medical, legal, and ethical standards.

KEY CONCEPTS

• Determining a dental hygiene diagnosis, formulating a treatment plan, and completely and accurately documenting all aspects of the dental hygiene process of care are elements of the standards for clinical dental hygiene practice.

- Identifying the goal of a case presentation, the intended audience and the significant aspects to include are elements of both written and oral case presentations.

RELEVANCE TO CLINICAL PRACTICE

Formulating the dental hygiene diagnosis (DHDx) involves a process of clinical decision-making that takes into consideration the patient's health history, oral health needs and values, and findings from assessment procedures. The dental hygienist uses these resources to determine existing or potential health problems that require further intervention. These patient problems become the basis for creating a treatment plan. The **treatment plan** delineates the treatment interventions that the dental hygienist and the patient will implement. Use of a DHDx provides the basis for individualized treatment plans that will help each patient achieve optimum oral and general health.

The Basics

1. Define the dental hygiene process of care.
   A. The ability to recognize or identify a disease.
   B. Interpreting clinical findings.
   C. An approach to clinical practice.
   D. Oral health improvement.

2. A definitive diagnosis can be defined as:
   A. A situation in which conditions have similar characteristics, signs, and symptoms.
   B. The identification or determination of a disease, problem, or injury.
   C. Listing in order of likelihood that those conditions or diseases may produce the signs observed.
   D. Conditions having similar characteristics, signs, and symptoms, and therefore a diagnosis cannot be readily determined.

3. According to the Dental Hygiene Process of Care (Fig. 18-1 in your textbook), assessment is considered:
   A. A framework where the individualized needs of the patient can be met.
   B. Identification of an individual's health behaviors.
   C. Establishment of goals and outcomes.
   D. Systematic collection, analysis, and documentation of the oral and general health status and patient needs.

4. Choose all that apply. Which of the following should be considered when developing a dental hygiene treatment plan?
   1) Assessment findings
   2) Patient's lifestyle
   3) Differential diagnosis
   4) Current scientific evidence
      A. 1, 2, and 3
      B. 1, 2, and 4
      C. 2, 3, and 4
      D. 1, 2, 3, and 4

5. All of the following conditions require a referral before dental hygiene treatment *except* for one. Which one is the *exception?*
   A. Uncontrolled diabetes
   B. Patient reports pain on tooth #30
   C. Blood pressure reading of 160/105 mm Hg
   D. Gingivitis associated with plaque biofilm

6. Choose the best description for the dental hygiene care plan.
   A. A thorough, individualized assessment of the person with or at risk for oral disease or complications.
   B. Complete and accurate recording of all collected data.
   C. List of interventions to promote the health or prevent disease of the patient's oral condition.
   D. The conscientious, explicit, and judicious use of current best evidence.

7. Which of the following is not part of the development of a treatment plan?
   A. The dental hygiene diagnosis must be determined before developing a treatment plan.
   B. The treatment plan should be comprehensive in addressing all of the patient's needs.
   C. The treatment plan should be problem-focused.
   D. The treatment plan should be patient-centered.

8. Match the term to the correct phrase as related to the four-prong approach to dental hygiene treatment planning.

   _____ Prevention   A. Home fluoride therapy

   _____ Treatment   B. Schedule an appointment to address caries

   _____ Maintenance   C. Perform CAMBRA

   _____ Referral   D. Evaluate for signs of candida infection and treat with antifungal medication

9. Explain how the dental hygienist determines a dental hygiene diagnosis.

   _____

   _____

   _____

10. List the 10 key elements for categorizing assessment information into the dental hygiene diagnosis.

    1) _____   6) _____

    2) _____   7) _____

    3) _____   8) _____

    4) _____   9) _____

    5) _____   10) _____

Learning Activities

1. Review a patient record from the dental hygiene clinic and critique the documented treatment plan. Determine whether or not the treatment plan was properly developed. Justify your conclusions. If improvements are needed, prepare a revised treatment plan and share it with your class.

2. Develop a dental hygiene treatment plan for a student partner. Present and critique the treatment plan in small groups.

Board Style Review Questions

1. The foundation for the dental hygiene diagnosis and treatment plan is derived from the:
   A. Assessment findings
   B. Diagnosis and prognosis
   C. Goals and expected outcomes
   D. Patient profile or demographics

2. Your patient arrives for his scheduled prophylaxis appointment and allows you to proceed with treatment. Based on his actions, this patient has provided:
    A. Articulated consent
    B. Expressed consent
    C. Implied consent
    D. Informed consent

3. Choose the component that represents dental hygiene treatment planning.
    A. Identifies tobacco history
    B. Assesses vital signs
    C. Compares blood pressure reading to previous readings
    D. Refers patient to the primary care physician for evaluation of elevated blood pressure

4. Choose the term that represents the identification of an existing or potential oral health problem that a dental hygienist is educationally qualified and licensed to treat.
    A. Differential diagnosis
    B. Dental hygiene diagnosis
    C. Dental hygiene process of care
    D. Standards of Clinical Dental Hygiene Practice

5. The diagnosis provides for:
    A. Evaluation strategies
    B. Goals and expected outcomes
    C. Risks and benefits of treatment
    D. Treatment rationale

6. Select the phrase that best describes the purpose of the dental hygiene diagnosis.
    A. To connect the differential diagnosis to a definitive diagnosis.
    B. To delineate the treatment interventions that the dental hygienist and the patient will implement.
    C. To provide a bridge between the assessment phase of care and the development of the treatment plan.
    D. To collaborate with the dentist.

7. If a clinician renders additional procedures without consent, the clinician could be libel for:
    A. Assault
    B. Battery
    C. Breach of contract
    D. Informed refusal

8. Choose the term that describes possible outcomes from the dental hygiene interventions that are performed for a patient.
    A. Treatment options
    B. Risks and benefits of treatment
    C. Dental hygiene prognosis
    D. Dental hygiene diagnosis

9. Identify the six components of the dental hygiene process of care.
    A. Assessment, dental hygiene diagnosis, planning, implementation, evaluation, and documentation.
    B. Assessment, consent, dental hygiene diagnosis, planning, implementation, and evaluation.
    C. Assessment, differential diagnosis, planning, implementation, evaluation, and documentation.
    D. Assessment, differential diagnosis, treatment plan, implementation, evaluation, and documentation.

10. The dental hygienist should record clinical information that subsequent providers can understand. This is a component of:
    1. Case presentation
    2. Consent
    3. Definitive diagnosis
    4. Documentation

Active Learning

Use the panoramic radiograph, the photograph, and the following information to answer these questions.

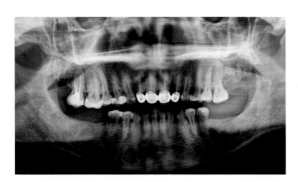 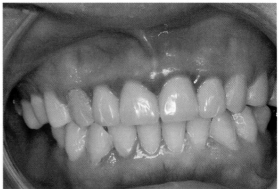

Patient profile: 32-year-old Asian female, works as a server, is married, has two children.
Medical history: No pertinent medical history, reports taking no medications, ASA I.
Dental history: Molars were extracted due to "cavities as a kid."
Chief complaint: I chew a lot of gum because my mouth is dry.
Oral hygiene assessment: Plaque score = 60%.

1. After analyzing and interpreting the provided assessment data, identify the dental hygiene diagnosis for this patient.
   A. Xerostomia
   B. Quadrant debridement with local anesthesia
   C. Medical consultation
   D. Patient education

2. Using the four-prong approach, develop a treatment plan for this patient.

   Prevention = _____

   Therapy = _____

   Maintenance = _____

   Referral = _____

3. Using the assessment data provided, what periodontal disease risk factors are evident?

   1) _____

   2) _____

   3) _____

   4) _____

Part VI

Treatment

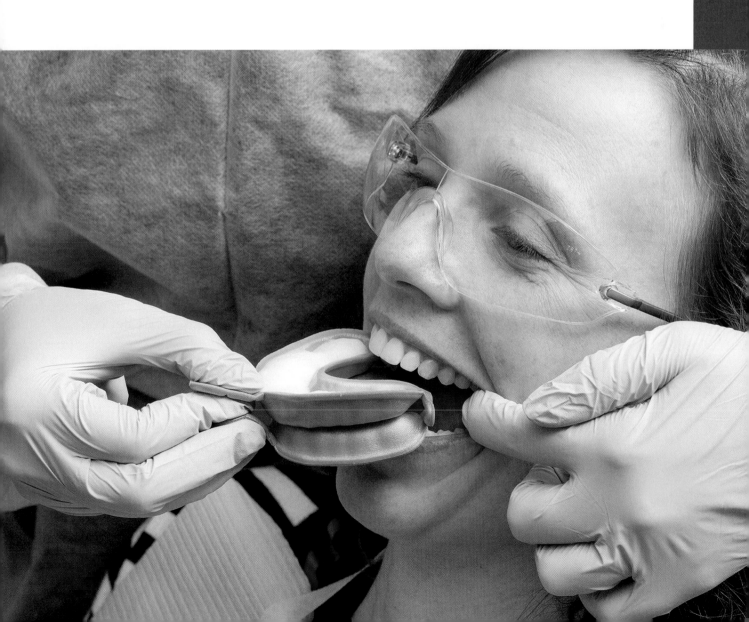

Chapter 19 | Devices

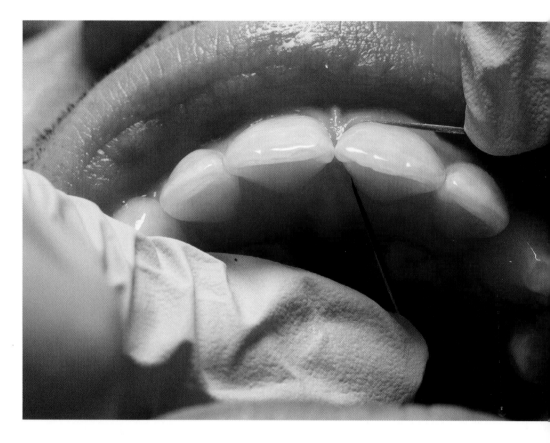

LEARNING OBJECTIVES

After reading this chapter, the student should be able to:

19.1 Discuss the role daily self-care plays in achieving and maintaining good oral health.

19.2 Explain the benefits and limitations of power and manual toothbrushes.

19.3 Compare and contrast the various types of interdental cleaning devices.

19.4 Recommend self-care devices to patients that are appropriate to their needs, interest, and ability.

19.5 Instruct a patient on how to use various types of self-care devices.

KEY CONCEPTS

• Tooth brushing is the primary and often only self-care habit utilized by most people.

• Interdental cleaning is needed by most patients to achieve good oral health.

• Successful recommendations include assessment of patient needs, ability, and interest, as well as instruction and education.

RELEVANCE TO CLINICAL PRACTICE

Daily self-care is critical to achieving and maintaining optimal oral health. The toothbrush is the most widely used self-care device, with 80% to 90% of people brushing one to two times per day.[1] Yet even the best-designed brushes cannot adequately clean between teeth, allowing for buildup of plaque biofilm. Most patients need some type of interdental cleaning. Compared with tooth brushing, only 10% to 30% of people use dental floss on a regular basis.[2]

The number and types of self-care options are larger today than ever. From manual and power toothbrushes to string floss, flossing aids/alternatives, interproximal brushes, toothpicks, and more for interdental cleaning, patients have a variety of choices (see Advancing Technologies). At the same time, the sheer volume of product offerings may confuse and overwhelm patients. One ideal product that can meet the needs of every patient does not exist. Dental hygienists play an important role in helping and motivating patients to find and use the product best suited for their unique situations. Table 19-1 shows how the recommendation of self-care devices fits into the dental hygiene process of care.

The Basics

1. Identify the product that can reduce subgingival bacteria in pockets up to 6 mm.
   - A. Interdental brush
   - B. Floss pick
   - C. Pulsating oral irrigator
   - D. Wood stick

2. How much plaque is removed by the average person who spends 1 min brushing?
   - A. 40%
   - B. 60%
   - C. 80%
   - D. 100%

3. What is the greatest advantage of the manual toothbrush?
   - A. Affordability
   - B. Design
   - C. Durability
   - D. Effectiveness

4. Your patient complains of food sticking between her teeth. Using this radiograph, choose the oral hygiene aids that are most appropriate for this patient.

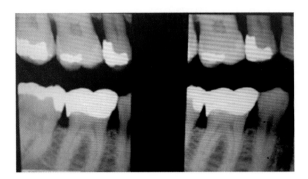

   1) Waxed floss
   2) Interdental brushes
   3) Water flosser
   4) Wood sticks
     A. 1 and 2
     B. 2 and 3
     C. 1, 2, and 4
     D. 2, 3, and 4

5. What is the ratio of chlorhexidine (CHX) to water in a 0.04% solution?
   A. 1 part CHX to 1 part water
   B. 1 part CHX to 2 parts water
   C. 1 part CHX to 3 parts water
   D. 1 part CHX to 4 parts water

6. All of your patients receive a manual toothbrush and dental floss at the end of their dental hygiene appointment. This practice may conflict with the self-care recommendations that you made during the appointment. What can you do differently to ensure that your actions support your recommendations?

_____

_____

7. How many people use dental floss on a regular basis?
   A. Less than 10%
   B. 10% to 30%
   C. 40% to 50%
   D. Greater than 50%

8. Match the process to the action.

   _____ Assessment   A. Identify how the patient will acquire a product.

   _____ Dental hygiene diagnosis   B. Answer questions for the patient about a product.

   _____ Planning   C. Use measurable criteria to determine the effectiveness of the procedure.

   _____ Implementation   D. Interpretation.

   _____ Evaluation   E. Verify embrasure size.

9. All of the following describe the Stillman or Modified Stillman tooth brushing method *except* for one. Which one is the *exception?*
   A. Appropriate choice for the patient who needs to massage or stimulate the gingiva.
   B. Filaments are place at a 45° angle toward the occlusal surfaces.
   C. The brush is placed part on the gingiva and part on the cervical area of the tooth.
   D. Pressure is applied to blanch the tissue.

10. Explain why gingivitis most readily starts in the col space.

_____

_____

_____

Learning Activities

1. Choose an oral health product from your local retail store. Prepare a 3 to 5 min presentation for your class. Include product device information such as cost, purpose, and evidence-based science to support the use of this product.

2. Discuss the factors to be considered when recommending a particular toothbrush.

_____

_____

_____

_____

Board Style Review Questions

1. Select the technique that directs the filaments of the toothbrush apically toward the teeth with the side of the brush on the attached gingiva.
   A. Bass
   B. Charters
   C. Modified Stillman
   D. Rolling stroke

2. Toothbrush bristles are generally identified as soft, medium, and hard. Soft toothbrushes have thicker and shorter bristles, whereas hard toothbrushes have bristles that are thinner and longer.
   A. Both statements are correct.
   B. The first statement is correct; the second statement is incorrect.
   C. Both statements are incorrect.
   D. The first statement is incorrect; the second statement is correct.

3. If an oral irrigation device with a classic jet tip is used, what is the expected depth of delivery in a 5 mm pocket?
   A. 44%
   B. 64%
   C. 68%
   D. 71%

4. Select the condition that would benefit the most from using the Charters method.
   A. Exposed cervical and proximal surfaces
   B. Gingival massage
   C. Gingival massage and stimulation
   D. Orthodontic appliances

5. Your patient has decided to start using a power toothbrush. What tooth brushing technique will you recommend?
   A. Bass
   B. Modified Stillman
   C. Rolling stroke
   D. The technique recommended in the manufacturer's instruction guide.

6. During the dental hygiene appointment, you are helping your patient choose a self-care device. Which of the following actions is _not_ part of the assessment process?
   A. Economic status
   B. Interest in the product
   C. Establishing a goal for how often the product is used
   D. Oral health status

7. The wood stick is traditionally made from all of the following materials *except* for one. Which one is the *exception?*
   A. Balsa
   B. Bass
   C. Beech
   D. Birch

8. The product that is most effective for unresolved gingivitis or bleeding is the:
   A. Wood stick
   B. Oral irrigator
   C. Interdental brush
   C. Dental floss holder

9. Your patient has good contact easement and a sulcus depth of 1 to 2 mm. Which product(s) are appropriate recommendations?
   1) Dental floss
   2) Dental floss holder
   3) Interdental brushes
   4) Wood sticks
      A. 1 and 2
      B. 2 and 3
      C. 2, 3, and 4
      D. 1, 2, 3, and 4

10. Identify the main disadvantage of the manual toothbrush.
    A. Cost
    B. Brush design
    C. Durability
    D. Efficacy is dependent on ability and technique

Active Learning

Mrs. Smith is a 40-year-old female who presents for a checkup and cleaning. She was diagnosed with multiple sclerosis and reports pain in her hands. Interpretation of her radiographs shows healthy bone levels and her periodontal probe depths range from 1 to 3 mm. While discussing her daily self-care routine, Mrs. Smith mentions that it is hard to hold her small toothbrush handle when her hands "flare up" and she does not use floss.

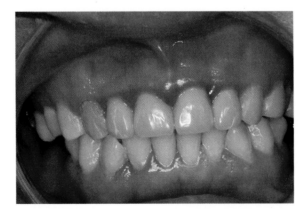

1. All of the following are assessment considerations for Mrs. Smith *except* for one. Which one is *not* a consideration for assessment of her daily self-care?
   A. Oral health status
   B. Manual dexterity
   C. Embrasure size
   D. Learning disabilities

2. Which of the following recommendations would you suggest for Mrs. Smith?
   1) Power toothbrush
   2) Add a tennis ball to a manual toothbrush handle
   3) Recommend more frequent recall appointments
   4) Rinse with chlorhexidine
      A. 2 and 3
      B. 3 and 4
      C. 1, 3, and 4
      D. 1, 2, 3, and 4

3. Select the device that is most appropriate for Mrs. Smith.
   A. Dental floss
   B. Interdental brushes
   C. Oral irrigator
   D. Wood sticks

REFERENCES

1. Van der Weijden GA, Timmerman MF, Danser MM, van der Velden U. The role of electric toothbrushes: advantages and limitations. In: Lang N, Attström R, Löe H, eds. *Proceedings of the European Workshop on Mechanical Plaque Control.* Chicago: Quintessence; 1998:138-155.
2. Berchier CE, Slots DE, Haps S, Van der Weijden GA. The efficacy of dental floss in addition to a toothbrush on plaque and parameters of gingival inflammation: a systematic review. *Int. J. Dent. Hyg.* 2008;6:265-279.

Chapter 20 | Dentrifices and Mouthrinses

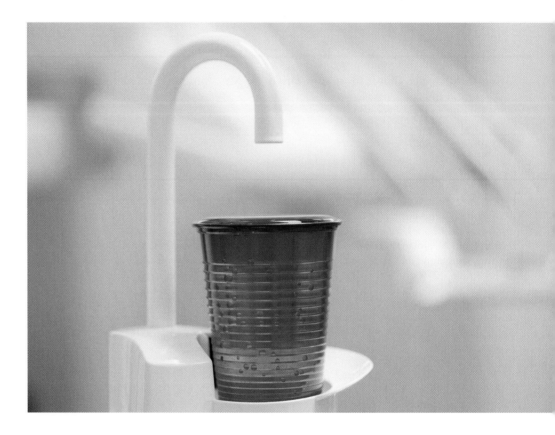

LEARNING OBJECTIVES

After reading this chapter, the student should be able to:

20.1 List and describe the basic ingredients of dentifrices and mouthrinses.

20.2 Select and recommend a dentifrice or mouthrinse for patients based on their needs.

20.3 Discuss the indications for use of different products based on their therapeutic ingredients.

20.4 Compare and contrast the active and inactive ingredients in dentifrices and mouthrinses.

20.5 Discuss potential adverse reactions for active and inactive ingredients in dentifrices and mouthrinses.

20.6 Identify key differences between prescription and over-the-counter dentifrices and mouthrinses.

20.7 Differentiate between the roles of the U.S. Food and Drug Administration and the American Dental Association in the regulation of dentifrices and mouthrinses.

KEY CONCEPTS

- Dentifrices and mouthrinses can be therapeutic adjuncts to brushing and flossing.
- An understanding of the different ingredients in dentifrices and mouthrinses can help the hygienist select the appropriate product to improve a patient's oral health.

RELEVANCE TO CLINICAL PRACTICE

Patients often ask their dental hygienist for information and advice regarding which toothpaste or mouthrinse would be the best choice for them. Substantial evidence supports the use of therapeutic dentifrices and/or mouthrinses as an adjunct to brushing and flossing. This chapter discusses common ingredients found in dentifrices and mouthrinses, and proper indications for their use. An understanding of the different ingredients in dentifrices and mouthrinses can help the dental hygienist recommend the appropriate product to improve a patient's oral health.

The Basics

1. All of the following are inactive ingredients in mouthrinse *except* for one. Which one is the *exception?*
   A. Alcohol
   B. Cetylpyridinium chloride
   C. Humectants
   D. Surfactants

2. Chlorhexidine gluconate is an ingredient used in mouthrinse to:
   1) Reduce gingivitis
   2) Whiten the teeth
   3) Reduce halitosis
   4) Clean/debride the teeth
      A. 1 and 2
      B. 1 and 3
      C. 1, 2, and 3

3. In the United States, dentrifices and mouthrinses are regulated by the:
   A. American Dental Association
   B. Food and Drug Administration
   C. National Institute of Health
   D. National Institute of Dental Research

4. Choose the correct statements related to toothpaste.
   1) The Food and Drug Administration assures the safety of both prescription and over-the-counter toothpastes.
   2) Cosmetic toothpastes must meet safety and therapeutic standards.
   3) Therapeutic toothpastes must meet safety guidelines.
   4) Therapeutic toothpastes require extensive documented testing for efficacy.
      A. 1 and 2
      B. 3 and 4
      C. 1, 3, and 4
      D. Only 4

5. Inactive ingredients help to maintain the toothpaste's consistency. Active ingredients provide therapeutic properties.
   A. Both statements are correct.
   B. The first statement is correct; the second statement is incorrect.
   C. Both statements are incorrect.
   D. The first statement is incorrect; the second statement is correct.

6. What percentage of the total toothpaste formulation is made up of thickening agents?
   A. 1% to 2%
   B. 3%
   C. 20% to 40%
   D. 20% to 60%

7. A reduction in calculus can result from:
   A. Reducing the pathogenicity of biofilm
   B. Chemical breakdown of stain pigments
   C. Decreasing nerve excitability
   D. Reducing crystal growth on the tooth surfaces

8. Identify the ingredient that suspends plaque and debris in an emulsion for easier removal during mechanical cleaning.
   A. Polishing agents
   B. Binders
   C. Humectants
   D. Surfactants

9. Choose the preservatives that prevent bacterial growth in toothpaste.
   1) Benzoates
   2) Parabens
   3) Phenolics
   4) Synthetic cellulose
      A. 1 and 2
      B. 2 and 3
      C. 3 and 4
      D. 1, 2, and 3

10. Select the ingredient that can contribute to the sweetness of toothpaste.
    A. Sorbitol
    B. Mineral colloids
    C. Benzoates
    D. Sodium *N*-lauryl sarcosinate

Learning Activities

1. Explain the proper use of mouthrinses.

_____

_____

_____

_____

_____

_____

_____

_____

_____

_____

2. List the factors that influence abrasiveness in toothpaste. _____

_____

_____

_____

_____

_____

3. Discuss the process for obtaining the ADA Seal of Acceptance for the various dental products.

_____

_____

_____

_____

_____

_____

_____

_____

_____

_____

_____

_____

_____

_____

_____

_____

_____

_____

Board Style Review Questions

1. An example of a surfactant is:
   A. Calcium carbonate
   B. Glycerol
   C. Seaweed colloids
   D. Sodium lauryl sulfate

2. All of the following are toothpaste abrasives/polishing agents *except* for one. Which one is the *exception?*
   A. Aluminum oxide
   B. Dehydrated silica gels
   C. Propylene
   D. Calcium carbonate

3. Select the toothpaste ingredient that prevents dehydration of the formulation.
   A. Humectants
   B. Surfactants
   C. Binders
   D. Abrasives

4. The purpose of alcohol in mouthrinse is to:
   1) Remove oral debris
   2) Inhibit crystallization around the opening of the mouthrinse container
   3) Prevent water loss
   4) Help solubilize other ingredients
      A. 1, 2, and 3
      B. 1 and 4
      C. 2 and 3
      D. only 4

5. Your patient asks for a recommendation for over-the-counter toothpaste to help reduce tooth sensitivity. Which ingredient should the toothpaste contain?
   A. Triclosan
   B. Essential oils
   C. Potassium nitrate
   D. Sodium citrate

6. In the United States, the maximum allowable fluoride in over-the-counter dentrifices is:
   A. 1000 ppm
   B. 1500 ppm
   C. 2000 ppm
   D. 2500 ppm

7. Identify the toothpaste ingredient that reduces calculus and is an antitartar.
   A. Papain
   B. Potassium nitrate
   C. Sodium monofluorophosphate
   D. Triclosan

8. All of the following are antigingivitis ingredients used in mouthrinse *except* for one. Which one is the *exception?*
   A. Benzocaine
   B. Cetylpyridinium chloride
   C. Chlorhexidine gluconate
   D. Essential oils

9. Select all of the ingredients that have been associated with extrinsic staining.
   1) Chlorhexidine gluconate
   2) Stannous fluoride
   3) Cetylpyridinium chloride
   4) Sodium monofluorophosphate
      A. 1, 2, and 3
      B. 1, 3, and 4
      C. 2 and 3
      D. 2 and 4

10. Which active ingredient should not be used frequently or for extended periods of time when the concentration is 3% or more in order to avoid damage to the oral tissues?
    A. Chlorine dioxide
    B. Hydrogen peroxide
    C. Terpene
    D. Thymol

Active Learning

Mr. Adam Wright presents for dental hygiene care. He is concerned with the staining of his teeth as seen in the photographs. He also asks for a recommendation for a mouthrinse for his bleeding gums. During your periodontal assessment, you discover that his tissue is red, spongy, smooth, and rolled. Use this information and the photographs to answer the following questions.

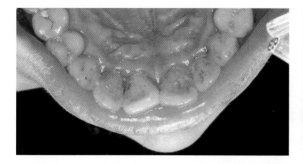 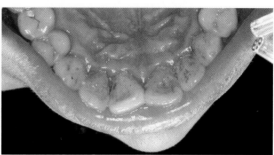

1. Based on the patient's chief concern, what ingredients in a toothpaste should the dental hygienist recommend for Mr. Wright?
   A. Calcium carbonate
   B. Dehydrated silica gels
   C. Glycerol
   D. Hydrated aluminum oxide

2. Based on the clinical assessments, what is the most appropriate ingredient in a mouthrinse to recommend for Mr. Wright?
   A. Chlorhexidine
   B. Polyvinylpyrrolidone
   C. Stannous fluoride
   D. Zinc salts

3. What contraindication should be considered when recommending chlorhexidine to this patient?

   _____

   _____

   _____

   _____

   _____

   _____

   _____

   _____

   _____

   _____

Chapter 21 | Cariology and Caries Management

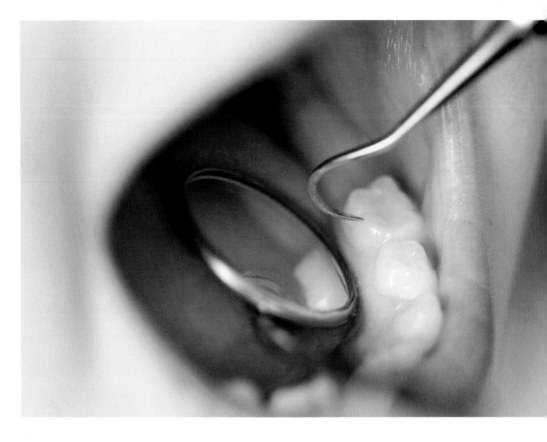

LEARNING OBJECTIVES

After reading this chapter, the student should be able to:

21.1 Discuss the most important distinctions among various terms used to describe the disease of mineralized structures.

21.2 Describe the multifactorial nature of the caries process.

21.3 Discuss the demineralization and remineralization processes and the importance of a balance between the two.

21.4 Explain the role fluoride and other preventive measures play in the remineralization process.

21.5 Describe how carious lesions are classified.

21.6 Discuss why early intervention using minimally invasive dentistry is critical to a therapeutic approach.

21.7 Identify the key elements of conducting a caries risk assessment.

21.8 Identify the specific primary risk factors and protective factors in the caries balance equation.

21.9 Explain how therapeutic recommendations differ among low-, moderate-, and high-risk status.

KEY CONCEPTS

- Caries is a multifactorial transmissible disease where cariogenic microorganisms interact in a dynamic relationship with factors that influence the disease process.
- The caries process can be reversed if it is identified in the early stages and protective factors are introduced.
- Fluoride is the primary therapeutic intervention in the prevention and control of caries.
- A caries risk assessment is essential in determining the level of risk and treatment protocols.
- A major paradigm shift to an interprofessional care model may help to identify, limit, and control oral diseases.

RELEVANCE TO CLINICAL PRACTICE

Current evidence reveals that the caries process exhibits a much more complex, multifactorial nature than was previously believed. Understanding the caries process has progressed from the early worm theory when barber surgeons hypothesized worms lived in the teeth and caused holes, to a research-based biological phenomenon.[1] Dental caries is a complex infectious disease process that afflicts 80% of the world's population. It is puzzling, though, how a largely preventable disease remains so prevalent.[1] New research is enhancing the understanding of the dynamic relationship among oral bacterial species, host dynamics, and measures that either promote or interfere with this disease process. Preventive regimens are key to minimizing caries risk and controlling the disease. Dental hygienists have expertise in designing and implementing preventive, oral, and nutritional education programs; they can effectively determine and recommend specific fluoride and nonfluoride caries preventive agents and recare intervals. Dental hygienists have the opportunity to take a leadership role in assisting patients to motivate themselves and in directing therapeutic care to decrease the burden of oral diseases and improve the quality of life for individuals and communities.

The Basics

1. Define cariology.
   A. Transmissible bacterial infectious disease process.
   B. End result of a dissolution of the tooth structure.
   C. The development of caries.
   D. Nontransmissible bacterial infectious disease process.

2. How many minutes does it take for the saliva to buffer the pH back to normal after a solid sugar exposure?
   A. 20 min
   B. 30 min
   C. 40 min
   D. 1 hr

3. All of the following glands produce saliva *except* for one. Which one is the *exception?*
   A. Parotid
   B. Sublingual
   C. Submandibular
   D. Submental

4. Extracellular polysaccharides store sucrose. Intracellular polysaccharides produce glucans.
   A. Both statements are correct.
   B. The first statement is correct; the second statement is incorrect.
   C. Both statements are incorrect.
   D. The first statement is incorrect; the second statement is correct.

5. Hydroxyapatite crystals begin to lose mineral content at a pH of:
   A. 5.0 to 5.5
   B. 6.5 to 6.7
   C. 7.0 to 7.2
   D. 7.5

6. All of the following are considered risk factors for dental caries *except* for one. Which one is the *exception?*
   A. Radiation therapy
   B. Visible white spots
   C. Heavy biofilm
   D. Saliva-reducing medications

7. How many minutes does it take for the saliva to buffer the pH back to normal after a liquid sugar exposure?
   A. 20 min
   B. 30 min
   C. 40 min
   D. 1 hr

8. Overall caries risk is determined by:
   A. Evaluating the number and severity of disease indicators and risk factors
   B. Adequacy of saliva flow
   C. Dietary habits
   D. Protective factors

9. List the protective factors of saliva.

_____

_____

_____

_____

_____

_____

_____

_____

_____

_____

_____

_____

_____

_____

10. Identify the incorrect statement for caries detection.
    A. Visual inspection can be used to assess for changes in color and surface texture of coronal surfaces.
    B. Digital fiber-optic transillumination can be used to detect incipient lesions.
    C. Tactile detection of coronal lesions with an explorer can be detrimental if excess pressure is used.
    D. Lesions detected on a radiograph are less advanced clinically than visible on a radiograph.

Learning Activities

1. Identify the two questions that have been validated for determining the frequency of consumption of liquids and snacks.

_____

_____

_____

_____

_____

_____

_____

_____

_____

_____

_____

_____

_____

_____

_____

_____

_____

_____

_____

_____

_____

_____

_____

2. Role-play with a student partner. Practice your dietary counseling technique.

Board Style Review Questions

1. Which phrase is incorrect in regards to the lactobacillus species?
   A. Increase in number in the later stages of lesion development
   B. Thrive in a very low pH environment
   C. Tend to displace other acidogenic bacteria
   D. Is one of the least acid-tolerant of the cariogenic microorganisms

2. Remineralized crystals are more acid-resistant due to:
   1) Higher carbonate content than hydroxyapatite crystals
   2) Fewer impurities
   3) Lower carbonate content than hydroxyapatite crystals
   4) More impurities
     A. 1 and 2
     B. 1 and 4
     C. 2 and 3
     D. 3 and 4

3. A loss of minerals in the oral cavity occurs when the pH drops less than:
   A. 5
   B. 5.5
   C. 7
   D. 14

4. The Caries Management by Risk Assessment protocol recommends that individuals at high risk:
   A. Rinse with 10 mL chlorhexidine 0.12% for 1 minute daily for 1 week each month
   B. Rinse with 5 mL chlorhexidine 0.12% for 30 seconds daily
   C. Rinse with 10 mL chlorhexidine 0.12% for 1 minute daily for 1 month
   D. Rinse with 5 mL chlorhexidine 0.12% for 1 minute twice daily for 1 week each month

5. Select the phrase that best describes the appearance of active enamel caries.
   A. Shiny with a smooth texture
   B. Chalky white with a smooth texture
   C. Shiny with a rough texture that may be white, yellow, brown, or black
   D. Chalky white with a matte or rough texture

6. Vertical transmission is:
   A. The presence of one or more decayed, missing of filled surfaces in any primary tooth in a child under the age of six.
   B. The acquisition of transmissible cariogenic microorganisms from a child's mother or primary caregiver.
   C. The acquisition of transmissible cariogenic microorganisms from a child's sibling.
   D. Special pattern of caries that differs from that found in older children.

7. Identify the *incorrect* phrase that relates to root caries.
   A. It occurs below the cementoenamel junction.
   B. A layer of biofilm covering the surface indicates activity of the lesion.
   C. Dissolution of cementum occurs less rapidly than with enamel caries.
   D. The texture is either soft and/or leathery.

8. Select all that apply to the radiographic detection of caries.
   1) Once a change in density is visible, the area is thought to be approximately 30% to 40% demineralized.
   2) Occlusal caries are generally moderate or advanced lesions before they are visible on radiographs.
   3) Radiographic sensitivity decreases as the lesion progresses toward the dentin.
   4) It is most effective when comparisons can be made with previous films.
     A. 1 and 2
     B. 1, 2, and 3
     C. 1, 2, and 4
     D. 2, 3, and 4

9. All of the following are true of fluoride varnish *except* for one. Which one is the *exception?*
   A. It is a resin base that is painted on the teeth to increase the contact time.
   B. It is available as an acidulated phosphate (APF) formula.
   C. It reduces the risk of ingestion compared with in-office gel products.
   D. It contains less fluoride than foam products.

10. Select the caries risk category for a patient who has any disease indicator for caries combined with a dry mouth.
    A. Low
    B. Moderate
    C. High
    D. Extreme

REFERENCES

1. Ruby JD, Cox, CF, Akimoto N. A review article. The caries phenomenon: a timeline from witchcraft and superstition to opinions of the 1500's to today's science. *Int J Dent.* 2010:1-10. doi:10.1155/2012/392730

Chapter 22 | Sealants

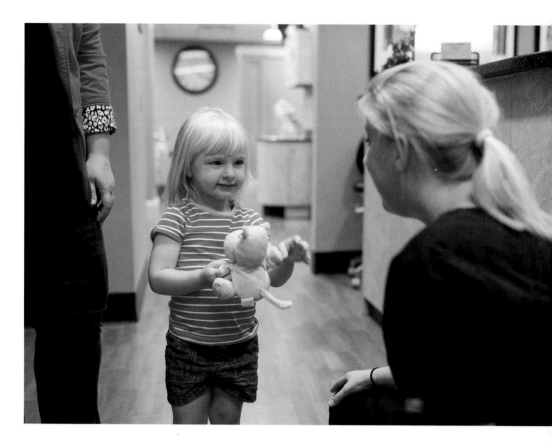

LEARNING OBJECTIVES

After reading this chapter, the student should be able to:

22.1 Discuss how sealants are part of an overall caries risk assessment and management protocol.

22.2 Outline the advantages and disadvantages of different types of sealants.

22.3 Successfully isolate a tooth in preparation for sealant placement.

22.4 Place a sealant and evaluate for retention.

22.5 Explain the sealant procedure to a patient.

KEY CONCEPTS

• Sealants are a primary way to prevent carious lesions in pits and fissures.

• Evaluation of sealants is a part of overall risk assessment.

• Proper technique and adherence to manufacturer's instructions are necessary for success in sealant placement.

RELEVANCE TO CLINICAL PRACTICE

Dental caries is the most common dental disease; it affects people of all ages. Five times more children have dental caries than asthma, hay fever, and chronic bronchitis combined. Eighty-five percent of adults have caries or have been treated for caries.[1] Caries is an infectious disease and, ironically, is preventable. Caries rates dropped drastically in the 1950s because of water fluoridation and increased use and awareness of the benefits of fluoride. Fluoride works best against smooth surface caries but does not always flow into the pits and fissures of teeth. It is well established that pit and fissure caries can be reduced by the placement of resin-based sealants. Studies show that reduction rates of caries range from 86% at 1 year to 58.6% at 4 years after placement.[2] It is crucial that dental hygienists be familiar with and skilled at the placement of dental sealants to effectively help their patients prevent oral disease.

The Basics

1. Describe a tooth that would benefit from a sealant.

_____

_____

_____

_____

_____

_____

_____

_____

_____

_____

_____

2. How would you describe the sealant process to a patient?

_____

_____

_____

_____

_____

_____

_____

_____

_____

_____

3. Obtain different types of sealants and classify them based on their polymerization process, filler content, color, and releasing properties.

Sealant/Brand	Polymerization process	Filler content	Color	Releasing properties

4. Describe situations when each of these sealants would be most beneficial to use.

_____

_____

_____

_____

_____

_____

_____

_____

_____

_____

5. Compare and contrast the conditions when a sealant is indicated or contraindicated.

_____

_____

_____

_____

_____

_____

_____

_____

_____

6. List the materials needed to place a sealant. Explain the function of each material during the sealant application process.

MATERIAL	FUNCTION
_____	_____
_____	_____
_____	_____
_____	_____
_____	_____
_____	_____
_____	_____
_____	_____
_____	_____
_____	_____
_____	_____
_____	_____

7. Describe scenarios when sealant placement might be compromised.

_____

_____

_____

_____

_____

_____

_____

_____

_____

_____

8. You completed a prophylaxis on a child, and the dentist suggests placing sealants on #2 and #3. How would you obtain informed consent? How would you document informed consent?

_____

_____

_____

_____

_____

_____

_____

_____

_____

_____

9. Use the case study from the textbook to assess the patient's caries risk using the systematic process for risk assessment (see Table 17-1 in the textbook).

Assessment
Analysis
Dental hygiene diagnosis
Plan
Implementation
Evaluation
Documentation

Learning Activities

1. Practice placing different types of sealants, and identify your errors.

_____

_____

_____

_____

_____

_____

2. Identify any errors on mounted teeth. Describe what caused the error. Describe how to correct the error.

_____

_____

_____

_____

_____

3. You have been asked to describe the rationale for sealants to pediatric nursing staff at a local hospital. Explain the rationale for placing sealants. Practice explaining this rationale to both allied health professionals and patients. Note any key differences.

_____

_____

_____

_____

_____

_____

4. You have placed sealants on all the first molars of a 6-year-old child. How would you document this in your treatment notes?

_____

_____

_____

_____

_____

Board Style Review Questions

1. From the following list, select the essential items needed for sealant placement.
   A. Acid etch
   B. Bite block
   C. Fluoride dentifrice
   D. Floss
   E. Articulating paper
   F. Explorer
   G. Mirror

2. Order the process of applying a sealant. Match each letter with its proper sequence number.

   _____ A. Assess with articulating paper

   _____ B. Apply acid etch per manufacturer's instructions

   _____ C. Clean the tooth surface

   _____ D. Rinse thoroughly and dry

   _____ E. Cure per the manufacturer's instructions

   _____ F. Apply sealant material

   _____ G. Dry tooth

   _____ H. Isolate tooth

   _____ I. Assess with explorer

3. From the following list, select the situations where sealant application would be contraindicated:
   A. Large occlusal restoration is present
   B. Caries on the interproximal surface
   C. Incipient caries lesion present in pit or fissure
   D. Open occlusal carious lesion present into dentin
   E. Patient wears bruxism appliance at night
   F. Patient has coalesced, shallow, or fused fissures

4. Obtaining informed consent for sealants is optional because sealants are usually placed on patients between the ages of 6 to 12.
   A. Both the statement and reason are correct and related.
   B. Both the statement and reason are correct but *not* related.
   C. The statement is correct; the reason is *not*.
   D. The statement is *not* correct; the reason is correct.
   E. *Neither* the statement *nor* the reason is correct.

5. Pits and fissures on permanent teeth can be U-shaped, V-shaped, Y-shaped, or Y2-shaped. Sealants are more effective on Y-shaped and Y2-shaped fissures than U-shaped or V-shaped fissures.
   A. Both statements are true.
   B. Both statements are false.
   C. The first statement is true; the second is false.
   D. The first statement is false; the second is true.

6. During a risk assessment, which factors are indications for sealant placement?
   1) Patient's salivary flow
   2) Patient's tooth anatomy
   3) Patient's recall interval
   4) Patient's caries risk
      A. 1 and 2
      B. 2 and 3
      C. 2 and 4
      D. 1, 2, and 4

7. Identify the materials that are added to sealants to increase durability and make them more resistant to wear.
   1) Amorphous calcium phosphate
   2) Fluoride
   3) Quartz
   4) Silica
      A. 1 and 2
      B. 1 and 3
      C. 2 and 4
      D. 3 and 4

8. Which of the following statements regarding four-handed delivery technique sealant placement is correct?
   A. Sealants should not be placed without an assistant.
   B. Hygienists should be able to place sealants both independently and with an assistant.
   C. The four-handed delivery approach has not been shown to improve the retention of sealants.
   D. The four-handed delivery technique should always be used when placing more than one sealant at a time in a quadrant.

9. How do sealants attach to the tooth surface?
   A. Chemical bond
   B. Mechanical bond
   C. Both A and B
   D. Retention groove
   E. Sealants are not attached/bonded to the tooth surface

10. Identify the equipment/material that provides the *best* isolation.
   A. Bite block
   B. Cotton rolls
   C. Dry angles
   D. Rubber dam

REFERENCES

1. U.S. Department of Health and Human Services. *Oral Health in America: A Report of the Surgeon General.* Rockville, MD: U.S. Department of Health and Human Services, National Institute of Dental and Craniofacial Research, National Institutes of Health, 2000.
2. Beauchamp J, Caufield PW, Crall JJ, et al. Evidence-based clinical recommendations for the use of pit-and-fissure sealants. *J Am Dent Assoc.* 2008;139:257-268.

Rubrics/Process Evaluations

Process Evaluation Template		
Pit and Fissure Sealants		
Evaluation Criteria	**Criteria Met? (Y/N)**	**Comments**
Appropriate patient for sealants		
All areas that would benefit from sealants identified		
Sealants incorporated into treatment plan		
Procedure explained to patient		
Informed consent obtained and documented		
Appropriate material and equipment		
Proper patient and operator position		
Cleaned tooth surface before conditioning		
Conditioned tooth with etch		
Rinsed etch for 30 sec		
Confined etching to surfaces being sealed		
Conditioned surface has a frosted white appearance		
Dry field maintained throughout procedure		
Appropriate amount of sealant material		
Sealant is smooth with no voids or irregularities		
Assessed sealant for retention with explorer		
Assessed occlusion with articulating paper		
Assessed contact areas with floss		
Occlusion checked and adjusted (as appropriate)		
Can identify errors (if placement is unsuccessful)		
Maintained proper infection control		
Applied professional fluoride application after sealant placement		
Postcare instructions provided to patient		

Chapter 23 | Prostheses and Appliances

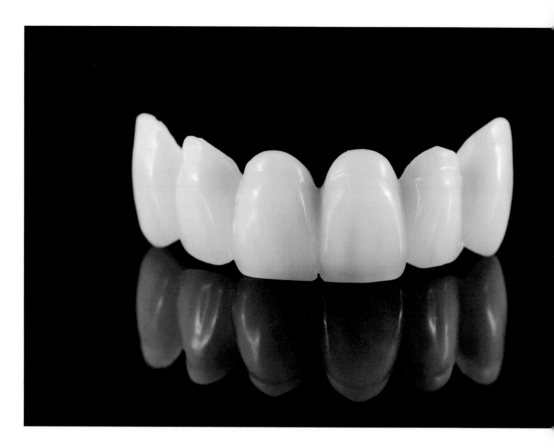

LEARNING OBJECTIVES

After reading this chapter, the student should be able to:

23.1 Describe the various ways missing teeth can be restored with fixed and removable prostheses.

23.2 Discuss the role dental implants play in replacing missing teeth.

23.3 Describe the various types of fixed and removable appliances used to influence the shape or function of the mouth and jaw.

23.4 Explain the importance of good oral hygiene, self-cleaning practices, and professional care for patients with prostheses and oral appliances.

23.5 Demonstrate appropriate self-care procedures for prostheses and oral appliances to a patient.

23.6 Discuss the necessary modifications in instrumentation for patients with implant-supported prostheses.

KEY CONCEPTS

• Missing teeth can be replaced with a variety of fixed and removable prostheses.

• Dental hygienists need to be familiar with all of the available treatment modalities for replacing missing teeth.

- Dental hygienists need to be familiar with the various types of fixed and removable oral appliances designed to influence the shape and function of the oral-facial structures.
- Prostheses and oral appliances require regular self-care and professional maintenance for optimal health and function.

RELEVANCE TO CLINICAL PRACTICE

The goal of modern dentistry is to restore individuals to optimal oral health in a predictable fashion regardless of oral disease, developmental defects, or injury to the oral and craniofacial system.[1] Millions of people in the United States alone experience dental caries, periodontal diseases, and anatomical defects such as cleft lip and palate. In 2004, more than 45% of adults in the United States, aged 65 years and older, were found to have six or more teeth missing.[2] Tooth loss caused by dental disease, congenital defects, and trauma affect an individual's ability to eat, swallow, and speak without discomfort, as well as her ability to maintain a healthy facial appearance. Malpositioned teeth and abnormal jaw relationships also influence an individual's ability to chew, eat, and speak, in addition to playing a role in the incidence of dental and periodontal infections and the individual's overall self-esteem. Oral disease caused by malignancies presents challenges in restoring function to the oral-facial structures. An estimated 30,000 cases of oral and pharyngeal cancers are diagnosed annually in the United States alone, creating a need for oral rehabilitation after surgical treatment.[3]

Dental hygienists must be well educated in the various treatment modalities and devices used in replacing missing oral structures, and they must recognize the various appliances that are designed to provide a therapeutic effect in the oral cavity. Dental hygienists must be able to educate patients regarding their treatment options and teach the appropriate self-care strategies. Dental hygienists must also be able to identify the materials used in oral prostheses and appliances, and apply the appropriate instrumentation principles for the professional care of these devices.

The Basics

1. All of the following are correct as related to the permucosal seal *except* for one. Which one is the *exception?*
   A. The permucosal seal is a soft tissue interface formed with the implant fixture and abutment.
   B. The permucosal seal is formed by the junctional epithelium.
   C. The permucosal seal protects from insults of bacterial plaque biofilm.
   D. The adjacent connective tissue contains more fibroblasts.

2. The supporting teeth in a fixed bridge are termed:
   A. Abutments
   B. Maryland bridge
   C. Overdenture
   D. Pontic

3. A fixed bridge designed to replace two missing teeth is called a:
   A. Double unit
   B. Two-unit bridge
   C. Four-unit bridge
   D. Pontic

4. Choose the best definition of osseointegration.
   A. Indirect biological attachment of living bone to a titanium implant surface without any intervening soft tissue.
   B. Direct biological attachment of living bone to a titanium implant surface with soft tissue intervention.
   C. Direct biological attachment of living bone to a titanium implant surface without any intervening soft tissue.
   D. Indirect biological attachment of living bone to a titanium implant surface with soft tissue intervention.

5. Dry, cracked epithelium at the corners of the mouth is a condition known as:
   A. Angular chelitis
   B. Denture stomatitis
   C. Edema
   D. Gingival hyperplasia

6. Implant configurations are:
   1) Angled
   2) Ball shaped
   3) Straight and conical
      A. 1 and 2
      B. 1 and 3
      C. 2 and 3
      D. 1, 2, and 3

7. What are the risks to not replacing a functioning tooth?
   1) Increased risk of periodontal infections.
   2) Migration of the opposing and adjacent teeth.
   3) Loss of alveolar bone due to lack of occlusal forces.
   4) Stress fractures.
      A. 1, 2, and 3
      B. 2 and 3
      C. 2, 3, and 4
      D. Only 2

8. List the key points for educating a patient with a removable oral prosthesis.

   1) _____

   2) _____

   3) _____

   4) _____

   5) _____

9. The dental hygienist should evaluate the abutment connection for:

   1) _____

   2) _____

   3) _____

10. What is a common problem associated with full dentures?

   _____

   _____

   _____

Learning Activities

1. Explain the importance of good oral hygiene practices for a patient with prosthesis and oral appliances.

   _____

   _____

   _____

   _____

2. Discuss appropriate instrumentation for patients with an implant-supported prosthesis.

   _____

   _____

   _____

   _____

Board Style Review Questions

1. The type of prostheses supported by retained natural roots or dental implants is called a(an):
   A. Complete denture
   B. Flipper
   C. Overdenture
   D. Removable partial denture

2. Titanium or gold-dipped instruments should be used for calculus removal on dental implants because the calculus that forms on dental implants is harder and more tenacious.
   A. The statement and the reason are correct.
   B. The statement is correct; the reason is incorrect.
   C. The statement and the reason are incorrect.
   D. The statement is incorrect; the reason is correct.

3. The portion of the implant that is screwed or tapped into the prepared bone is the:
   A. Abutment
   B. Fixture
   C. Prosthesis
   D. Superstructure

4. Which of the following is not a recommendation for daily prosthesis care?
   A. Place a small cloth in the sink.
   B. Brush the outer and inner surfaces of the prosthesis.
   C. Brush with a mild liquid soap.
   D. Rinse with hot water.

5. Choose the factors that can contribute to denture stomatitis.
   1) Allergic stimuli
   2) Bacteria
   3) Mechanical
   4) Viral
      A. 1 and 2
      B. 2 and 4
      C. 1, 2, and 3
      D. 1, 2, 3, and 4

6. The part of the endosteal implant that is located subgingivally within the peri-implant crevice is:
   A. Abutment
   B. Fixture
   C. Prosthesis
   D. Superstructure

7. Identify the correct phrases related to dental implants.
   1) Probing depths should be assessed regularly during the first 3 months of implant placement.
   2) Chlorhexidine gluconate is useful during the postsurgical healing phase.
   3) Radiographic interpretation can be used to assess the success or failure of an implant.
      A. 1 and 2
      B. 2 and 3
      C. 1, 2, and 3
      D. Only 1

8. Select the type of dental implant that is placed into the alveolar bone of the mandible or maxilla.
   A. Endosteal
   B. Subcutaneous
   C. Subperiosteal
   D. Transosteal

9. Choose the statement that best describes an obturator.
   A. It is designed to replace a single missing tooth.
   B. It is inflammation of the underlying soft tissues.
   C. It is designed to close a defect.
   D. It is a direct biological attachment of bone to implant surface.

10. Peri-implant mucositis is an inflammatory reaction in the hard and soft tissues. Peri-implantitis is a reversible, inflammatory reaction.
    A. Both statements are correct.
    B. The first statement is correct; the second statement is incorrect.
    C. Both statements are incorrect.
    D. The first statement is incorrect; the second statement is correct.

Active Learning

1. The condition observed in the photograph is classified as:

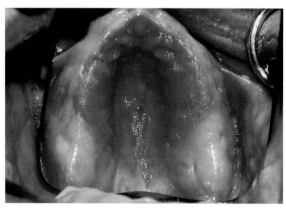

Photo courtesy of Phillip Dunn, DDS

   A. *Candida albicans*
   B. Denture stomatitis
   C. Lichen planus
   D. Peri-implantitis

2. This condition most likely occurred because the patient:
   A. Wears an overdenture
   B. Wears an obturator
   C. Wears a fixed prosthetic
   D. Wears a removable prosthetic

3. This patient most likely:
   1) Has a history of cleft palate
   2) Was diagnosed with a pharyngeal cancer
   3) Suffers from traumatic lesions
   4) Suffers with opportunistic fungal infections
      A. 2 and 3
      B. 2 and 4
      C. 3 and 4
      D. Only 1

REFERENCES

1. Misch CE. *Contemporary Implant Dentistry.* 3rd rev.ed. St Louis, MO: Mosby; 2007.
2. Centers for Disease Control and Prevention. National Oral Health Surveillance System. http://www.cdc.gov/nohss/index.htm. Accessed February 21, 2010.
3. U.S. Department of Health and Human Services (HHS). *Oral Health in America: A Report of the Surgeon General.* Rockville, MD: HHS, National Institutes of Health, National Institute of Dental and Craniofacial Research; 2000.

Rubrics/Process Evaluations

Process Evaluation Template

Cleaning a Removable Prosthesis/Appliance

Evaluation Criteria	Criteria Met? (Y/N)	Comments
Student wears appropriate PPE.		
Student asks patient to remove prosthesis.		
Student places prosthesis into a cup or small plastic bag and transfers to dental laboratory setting.		
Student places several paper towels in sink.		
Student uses a new or sterile brush to dislodge visible debris.		
Labels a self-locking plastic bag with the patient's name.		
Carefully rinses the prosthesis or appliance.		
Places the prosthesis or appliance in a self-locking plastic bag.		
Student selects an appropriate cleaning solution and adds to bag.		
Student places sealed bag into a small beaker filled with water. The beaker is immersed into an ultrasonic cleaner.		
Processes for appropriate amount of time.		
Student removes prosthesis or appliance from the bag and inspects for residual deposits and stains.		
Additional instrumentation implemented if required.		
Student returns denture to patient.		
Documentation completed.		

Chapter 24 | Ergonomics

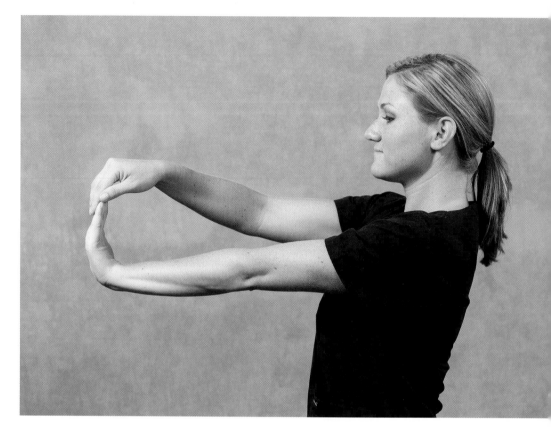

LEARNING OBJECTIVES

After reading this chapter, the student should be able to:

24.1 Define musculoskeletal disorders.

24.2 Define ergonomics.

24.3 State at least three common symptoms of musculoskeletal disorders.

24.4 Discuss the importance of an anteverted pelvis while performing clinical dental hygiene.

24.5 Describe at least two ways to open the pelvic angle while sitting.

24.6 Provide reasons to exercise while in the dental operatory.

24.7 Demonstrate one exercise each for the hands, neck, shoulders/upper trunk, back, and legs.

24.8 Explain why loupes and proper lighting are important for the dental hygienist.

24.9 List three aspects of instrument selection.

24.10 Explain four key concepts of instrumentation related to hand health.

KEY CONCEPTS

• Most musculoskeletal disorders (MSD) are insidious, but with applied knowledge about work environment (ergonomics), equipment adjustment, and patient and operator positioning, cumulative disorders can be minimized.

• Prevention of MSD occurs because risk factors are minimized or eliminated.

- An anteverted pelvis helps the body stay in a more upright position.
- Properly standing, sitting, and moving around the patient can help prevent musculoskeletal injuries.
- Chairside exercises, when done regularly and frequently, allow the clinician to work more comfortably and effectively.

RELEVANCE TO CLINICAL PRACTICE

Dental hygienists often complain about pain in their hands, arms, neck, shoulders, and upper and lower back. Clinically, these pains describe **musculoskeletal disorders (MSD)**. These disorders are not the result of a single event but develop over time from the chronic use of repetitive, forceful, and awkward movements or postures at work or at home.[1] Affected areas include the soft tissues of the body, including nerves, tendons, and muscles. Symptoms may include pain, swelling, burning sensations, cramping, decreased range of motion, stiffness, muscle weakness, tingling, and numbness.

Studies regarding MSD among dental hygiene students are quite limited; however, musculoskeletal problems have become a significant issue for the profession of dentistry, including dental hygiene, and represent a significant burden. Factors that contribute to pain among dental professionals include poorly designed workstations, inadequate equipment, inappropriate work patterns, repetitive work, neck flexion, upper arm abduction, prolonged static postures, awkward positioning, and precise motions.[2] The key to preventing MSD is to minimize risk factors.

The Basics

1. Standing is the ideal position for the clinician when treating the maxillary arch. The dental hygienist can vary his/her posture by sitting while treating the mandibular arch.
   A. Both statements are correct.
   B. The first statement is correct; the second statement is incorrect.
   C. Both statements are incorrect.
   D. The first statement is incorrect; the second statement is correct.

2. Identify the most important operatory/office exercise.
   A. Lateral trunk stretch
   B. Neck stretches
   C. Navel in and up
   D. Wrist flexor and extensor stretch

3. When selecting hand instruments that will be used for extended periods of time, the handles that are the least beneficial are:
   A. Smaller or thinner handles
   B. Round handles
   C. Hollow or resin handles
   D. Textured handles

4. Leaning forward toward a patient can lead to:
   1) Shortening and tightening of the muscles on the front of the body.
   2) Weakening and elongation of the muscles on the back of the body.
   3) Impaired breathing.
      A. 1 and 2
      B. 1 and 3
      C. 2 and 3
      D. 1, 2, and 3

5. Choose the best definition for dynamic sitting.
   A. Saddle-shaped seating
   B. Alternating between half standing and sitting
   C. Chair position that reduces muscle strain and decreases intervertebral disk pressure.
   D. Position that allows the hygienist to sit up with the tailbone back.

6. Select the best solution for trunk twisting.
   A. Elongate the spinal column
   B. Align the trunk vertically
   C. Preserve anterior version of pelvic girdle
   D. Use chair castors to allow for easier turning

7. List the benefits to standing while performing clinical dental hygiene.

   1) _____
   _____

   2) _____
   _____

   3) _____
   _____

   4) _____
   _____

   5) _____
   _____

   6) _____
   _____

8. Choose the term for the scientific discipline of interactions among humans and other elements that optimize human well-being and overall system performances.
   A. Musculoskeletal disorders
   B. Ergonomics
   C. Trigger points
   D. Anterior version pelvic position

9. Explain why sharp instruments are so important.

   _____
   _____
   _____
   _____
   _____
   _____
   _____

10. List three considerations for selecting a headlight.

1) _____

_____

_____

2) _____

_____

_____

3) _____

_____

_____

Learning Activities

1. Explain what can happen if one hip is off center.

_____

_____

_____

_____

_____

_____

_____

_____

2. Describe the benefits of using magnification loupes.

_____

_____

_____

_____

_____

_____

_____

Board Style Review Questions

1. Which condition can lead to a lazy or clumsy hand?
   A. Carpal tunnel syndrome
   B. Myofascial pain syndrome
   C. Rotator cuff problems
   D. Thoracic outlet syndrome

2. Identify the *incorrect* statement related to anterior version pelvic position.
   A. Elbows should be lower than the shoulders.
   B. Wrists should be slightly higher than the elbows.
   C. The dental hygienist should lean in from the waist.
   D. Keep the forearm parallel to the floor.

3. When treating the maxillary arch, the patient's occlusal plane should be parallel to the floor. For treatment of the mandibular arch, the patient's occlusal plane should be positioned perpendicular to the floor.
   A. Both statements are true.
   B. The first statement is true; the second statement is false.
   C. Both statements are false.
   D. The first statement is false; the second statement is true.

4. Almost every syndrome or condition stems from:
   A. An anteverted pelvis
   B. Keeping the back straight
   C. Leaning, twisting, and reaching
   D. Improper seating

5. The ilium should be positioned forward of the ischial tuberosities. This allows the dental hygienist to sit up with the coccyx positioned back.
   A. Both statements are correct.
   B. The first statement is correct; the second statement is incorrect.
   C. Both statements are incorrect.
   D. The first statement is incorrect; the second statement is correct.

6. To open the pelvis, the dental hygienist can:
   1) Decrease the chair height
   2) Increase the chair height
   3) Keep the hips slightly higher than the knees
   4) Keep the hips slightly lower than the knees
      A. 1 and 3
      B. 1 and 4
      C. 2 and 3
      D. 2 and 4

7. To keep the hips in anteversion, the angle of the hips needs to be between:
   A. 50° to 90°
   B. 90° to 110°
   C. 110° to 130°
   D. Greater than 130°

8. To prevent hand problems it is recommended that the dental hygienist choose:
   A. Only large diameter instruments
   B. Vary handle size
   C. Use only textured instruments
   D. Use only thinner handles

9. All of the following are correct descriptions of loupes *except* for one. Which one is the *exception?*
   A. They increase field size.
   B. They allow for improved posture with correct focal length and declination angle.
   C. They increase brightness.
   D. They decrease field size.

10. Identify the unhealthy working position/posture.
    A. Trunk laterally flexed
    B. Spinal column is elongated
    C. Feet are flat on the floor and positioned apart
    D. Arms are placed by side near rib cage

REFERENCES

1. Hamann C, Werner R, Rhode N, Rogers P, Sullivan K. Upper extremity musculoskeletal disorders in dental hygiene: diagnosis and options for management. *Contemp Oral Hyg.* 2004;4:2-8.
2. Hayes M, Cockrell D, Smith D. A systematic review of musculoskeletal disorders among dental professionals. *Int J Dent Hyg.* 2009;7(3):159-165.

Rubrics/Process Evaluations

Process Evaluation Template		
Ergonomics		
Evaluation Criteria	**Criteria Met? (Y/N)**	**Comments**
The student...		
Positions the patient so that the clinician's elbows are lower than the shoulders.		
Keeps the neck as vertical as possible.		
Keeps shoulders horizontal (not lifted or hunched).		
Leans from the waist-in; "ready" position.		
Keeps upper arms parallel to the torso with elbows at waist level.		
Maintains thumb slightly higher than the little finger and wrist is aligned with the forearm.		
Positions the back of the chair forward during treatment of the mandibular arch so that the occlusal plane is parallel to the floor.		
Positions the back of the chair as far back as possible during treatment of the maxillary arch so that the occlusal plane is perpendicular to the floor.		
Keeps his/her arms by the sides, near the ribcage.		
Feet are apart and flat on the floor		
Alternates between sitting and standing.		
Uses properly fitted loupes.		
Uses properly fitted gloves.		
Follows standard precautions.		

Chapter 25 | Power Scaling

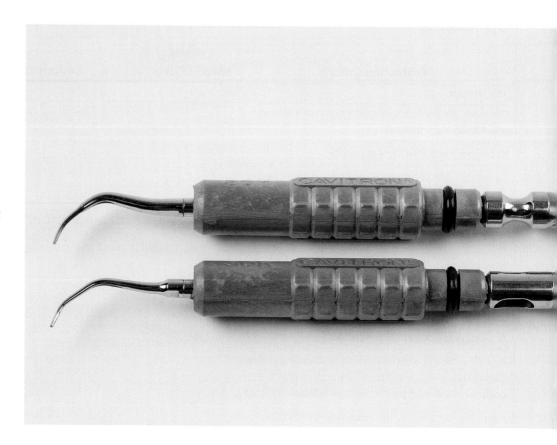

LEARNING OBJECTIVES

After reading this chapter, the student should be able to:

25.1 Discuss the principles and mechanisms of action for powered scaling devices.

25.2 Describe the types of power scaling devices that are available.

25.3 Understand and explain the advantages and disadvantages of power scaling compared with manual instrumentation.

25.4 Identify appropriate inserts/tips for use in a variety of clinical circumstances.

25.5 Describe the proper activation and care of ultrasonic inserts.

KEY CONCEPTS

• Power scaling can effectively treat a wide range of patient needs from maintaining oral health to treating patients with periodontal disease.

• Power scaling is an efficient and effective means for full-mouth debridement.

• Proper technique and tip selection is necessary for success in thorough debridement.

RELEVANCE TO CLINICAL PRACTICE

Power scaling has been used for periodontal procedures for more than 50 years and will continue to be used in the future. The evolution of power scaling devices and inserts has been tremendous. Due to current research findings regarding the pathogenesis of periodontal disease, power scaling can and should be used on nearly every patient undergoing periodontal debridement procedures, including routine visits for recare, periodontal maintenance, and periodontal therapy. New technology has allowed researchers to discover that bacterial plaque is sophisticated and exists as complex matrices called *biofilms*.[1] The only way to improve periodontal health is to remove or disrupt the biofilm.[2] This can be accomplished effectively with manual instrumentation or power scaling devices, but there are advantages when power scaling is used.

The Basics

1. The unit of energy that measures cycles per second is called:
   A. Amplitude
   B. Frequency
   C. Hertz (Hz)
   D. Milliamps

2. Ultrasonic power scaling devices operate at a frequency of:
   A. 3000 to 8000 cps
   B. 18,000 to 50,000 cps
   C. 25 K
   D. 30 K

3. Triple-bend tips are designed for:
   A. Heavy to gross debridement
   B. Interproximal surfaces of posterior teeth
   C. Enhanced access in periodontal pockets
   D. Malpositioned and concave surfaces

4. Select the phrases that describe sonic scalers.
   1) Uses a self-contained electronic generator
   2) Activated by a foot pedal attached to the dental unit
   3) Connects to the dental unit's compressed air valve
   4) Activated by a foot pedal attached to the power scaling device
      A. 1 and 2
      B. 1 and 4
      C. 2 and 3
      D. 3 and 4

5. Select the power scaling device that uses tips that alternate electrical currents applied to crystals.
   A. Magnetostrictive
   B. Piezoelectric
   C. Sonic

6. A fulcrum too close to the working surface of the tooth may disrupt a balanced ultrasonic grasp; therefore, the dental hygienist should consider using an alternate or advanced fulcrum.
   A. Both the statement and the reason are correct.
   B. The statement is correct; the reason is incorrect.
   C. Both the statement and the reason are incorrect.
   D. The statement is incorrect; the reason is correct.

7. All of the following are correct as related to adaptation for power scaling *except* for one. Which one is the *exception?*
   A. Keep the terminal 2 to 3 mm of the tip adapted against the tooth.
   B. Keep the tip moving.
   C. Start with the highest power setting for maximum effectiveness.
   D. Use overlapping vertical, horizontal, and oblique strokes.

8. Match the appropriate tip to the task.

   _____ Beaver-tail tip   A. Universal tip designed for heavy to gross deposit removal.

   _____ Bladed tip   B. Debridement of periodontal pockets with light to medium deposits.

   _____ Diamond-coated tip   C. Universal tip for debridement of heavy buccal and lingual deposits.

   _____ Triple-bend tip   D. Debridement of light to heavy supragingival calculus in shallow pockets.

9. The 0.08 mm ball at the end of an ultrasonic tip is used to:
   A. Allow the instrument to swivel
   B. Prevent gouging in the furcation area
   C. Detect entry into a furcation
   D. To instrument concave surfaces

10. Identify the tip that is most effective on interproximal surfaces of posterior teeth, tight contact areas, and malpositioned teeth.
    A. Triple-bend tips
    B. Straight tips
    C. Beaver-tail tips
    D. Curved right and left tips

Learning Activities

1. Discuss the advantages of power scaling devices.

_____

_____

_____

_____

_____

_____

_____

_____

_____

_____

_____

_____

_____

_____

_____

_____

_____

2. Explore the various inserts/tips available at your clinical setting. Identify the inserts by name and use.

3. Evaluate the ultrasonic inserts for wear. Describe proper maintenance of inserts/tips.

_____

_____

_____

_____

_____

_____

_____

_____

_____

_____

_____

_____

_____

_____

_____

_____

_____

Board Style Review Questions

1. The term frequency can be defined as:
   A. Rapid movement of air bubbles from the tip of the insert.
   B. Small currents in the water.
   C. The distance the tip moves.
   D. The number of times an instrument tip vibrates.

2. Which power scaling device has the lowest frequency?
   A. Magnetostrictive units
   B. Piezoelectric units
   C. Sonic scalers
   D. Ultrasonic scalers

3. All of the following are correct of piezoelectric units _except_ for one. Which one is the _exception?_
   A. Tips screw into a handpiece with a wrench-type device
   B. Tips work in a linear motion
   C. Little heat is generated
   D. All sides of the working tip can be used

4. Choose the best definition for cavitation.
   A. Rapid movement of air bubbles from the tip of the insert.
   B. Small currents in the water.
   C. The distance the tip moves.
   D. The number of times an instrument tip vibrates.

5. A higher power setting delivers a shorter stroke. A lower power setting delivers a longer stroke.
   A. Both statements are correct.
   B. The first statement is correct; the second statement is incorrect.
   C. Both statements are incorrect.
   D. The first statement is incorrect; the second statement is correct.

6. The distance the tip moves or the length of the stroke is called:
   A. Amplitude
   B. Frequency
   C. Hertz (Hz)
   D. Lavage

7. Select the tip that provides better access to deeper periodontal pockets.
   A. Beavertail
   B. Slim
   C. Standard
   D. Universal

8. Piezoelectric units operate at a higher frequency than magnetostrictive units. Piezoelectric units use more water than magnetostrictive units because more heat is generated.
   A. Both statements are true.
   B. The first statement is true; the second statement is false.
   C. Both statements are false.
   D. The first statement is false; the second statement is true.

9. All of the following are contraindications for using power scaling devices *except* for one. Which one is the *exception?*
   A. Patient with known communicable disease.
   B. Periodontal debridement procedures requiring only deplaquing.
   C. Areas of demineralization.
   D. Patients with older model pacemakers.

10. Choose the tip that is best for removal of moderate to heavy calculus deposits.
    A. Diamond-coated
    B. Slim
    C. Periodontal
    D. Universal

REFERENCES

1. Overman P. Biofilm: A new view of plaque. *J Contemp Dent Pract.* 2000;1(3):18-29.
2. Sbordone L, Ramaglia L, Gulletta E, Iacono V. Recolonization of the subgingival microflora after scaling and root planing in human periodontitis. *J Periodontol.* 1990;61(9):579-584.

Rubrics/Process Evaluations

Process Evaluation Template		
Power Scaling		
Evaluation Criteria	**Criteria Met? (Y/N)**	**Comments**
The student. . .		
Flushes waterline to the power scaling device for 2 to 3 minutes.		
Selects appropriate tip.		
Fills handle with water before inserting tip on magnetostrictive units.		
Directs patient to complete a 30 sec preprocedural rinse with an antimicrobial solution.		
Informs patient that a power scaling device will be used for debridement.		
Places the patient in a supine position.		
Utilizes a balanced grasp and light lateral pressure.		
Wraps the cord around forearm or between fingers to reduce tension and torque.		
Establishes ideal intraoral or extraoral fulcrum.		
Keeps the terminal 2 to 3 mm of the tip adapted and moving at all times.		
Starts at the lowest effective power setting.		
Follows sequence of inserting the tip subgingivally at the distal line angle, moves toward contact (across the interproximal surface).		
Reinserts tip at the distal line angle and moves across the facial or lingual surface to the mesial line angle through to the mesial proximal surface.		
Uses appropriate fluid evacuation.		
Evaluates effectiveness of procedure with the explorer.		
Properly documents procedure including patient's tolerance.		
Uses standard precautions during procedure.		

Chapter 26 | Instrumentation Principles and Techniques

KEY TERMS

adaptation

angulation

curettage

digital motion activation

file

fulcrum

handle rolling

hoe

motion activation

pivoting

universal instruments

wrist motion activation

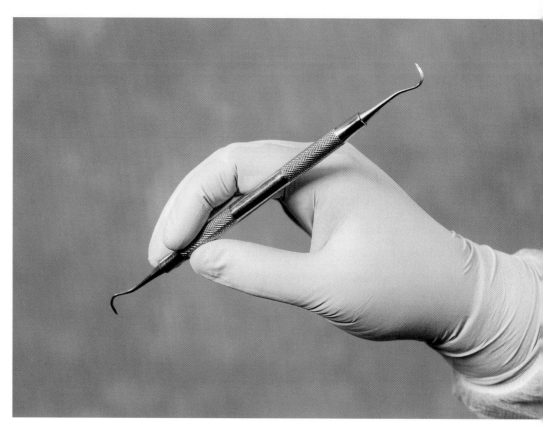

LEARNING OBJECTIVES

After reading this chapter, the student should be able to:

26.1 Use the modified pen grasp in practice.

26.2 Differentiate among the three parts of the working end of the curet and sickle scaler.

26.3 Adapt the working end of the anterior sickle scaler.

26.4 Demonstrate the process of inserting the working end of the sickle and curet into the sulcus or beneath the gingival margin.

26.5 Apply the appropriate working end of a universal curet to the distal surface of a mandibular posterior tooth.

26.6 Demonstrate the correct angulation of the instrument for the process of calculus removal.

26.7 Demonstrate wrist motion activation.

26.8 Demonstrate hand pivot and handle roll.

26.9 Use proper technique to stabilize the hand and instrument to perform an instrumentation stroke.

26.10 Use the correct techniques for instrument sharpening.

KEY CONCEPTS

- The major conventional methods for removing biofilm, calculus, and altered cementum are scaling and root planing.
- Risk evaluation includes the assessment of tissue healing patterns and pocket depth rates.
- The success of periodontal therapy is linked to the effectiveness of scaling and root planing.
- The success of treatment of patients with gingivitis and periodontitis in early stages depends on several factors, among them efficient patient education, recognition of the disease, and appropriate instrumentation.

RELEVANCE TO CLINICAL PRACTICE

Evidence-based care defines instrumentation for the processes of calculus and biofilm removal and ensures that treatment is optimum. Periodontal debridement (previously restricted to scaling and root planing) is essential to periodontal health for the following reasons:

1. It blocks the development of periodontal diseases through physical removal of biofilm and calculus deposits.
2. It creates a healthy environment that assists in keeping tissues intact and allows the gingival tissue to be restored, reducing and removing inflammation.
3. It contributes to better oral self-care by providing healing in those potentially disease-causing areas that patients cannot access themselves.[1]

This technique is also referred to as nonsurgical periodontal therapy. In general, it presupposes the removal of supragingival and subgingival deposits of calculus and biofilm. This procedure is technically challenging, and its efficiency is bound to the depth of the pocket, skill of the dental hygienist, anatomy of the root, time spent, and sharpness of instruments. Scaling and root surface debridement are normally conducted with the help of hand instruments and sonic or ultrasonic instruments. Traditional therapy is given during a series of appointments. Full-mouth disinfection may be used to reduce the risk of healing pockets being re-infected; the treatment is completed within 24 hours. However, systemic or local factors, as well as the technical aspect of the work, may restrict the effectiveness of this type of therapy. In this case, surgical approaches or adjunctive antimicrobials are used.[2]

The terms *scaling* and *root planing* were widely used in the past. *Scaling* is the removal of hard and soft deposits from the crown and root surfaces whereas *root planing* is defined as the removal of cementum and dentin that is impregnated with bacteria, endotoxins, and calculus.[3] The dental hygiene field uses the term *periodontal debridement*, because it presupposes preservation of cementum for a faster and more efficient healing process in patients. It also concentrates on the removal of calculus and bacteria biofilm from root and crown surfaces, but attempts to leave cementum intact. Because of the superficial association of endotoxin and cementum, it is unnecessary to remove the cementum, given the undesirable side effects such as pulpitis and hypersensitivity that may result from its removal.[4]

The Basics

1. The convergence of the two lateral surfaces with the face of an instrument is termed the:
    A. Back
    B. Cutting edge
    C. Face
    D. Tip

2. What degree of angulation is needed for calculus removal/scaling stroke?
    A. 0 to 40
    B. 50 to 70
    C. 60 to 70
    D. 70 to 80

3. Identify the type of shank of a sickle scaler.
    A. Inflexible
    B. Flexible
    C. Moderately flexible
    D. Rigid

4. In a modified pen grasp, which fingers hold the instrument handle?
    1) Index finger
    2) Middle finger
    3) Ring finger
    4) Thumb
        A. 1 and 2
        B. 1 and 4
        C. 2 and 3
        D. 3 and 4

5. The portion of the instrument that covers the area from the working end of the instrument to the bend closest to the handle is the:
    A. Functional shank
    B. Lower shank
    C. Terminal shank
    D. Working end

6. What component of the instrument determines its function?
    A. Handle
    B. Shank
    C. Tip
    D. Working end

7. The cutting edges of a sickle scaler converge to form the:
    A. Back
    B. Face
    C. Tip
    D. Toe

8. Match the instrument type to the best descriptor.

_____ Anterior sickle	A. Complex shank
_____ File	B. Single cutting edge created by the connection of the beveled toe and face of the blade
_____ Hoe	C. Straight blade, shank, and handle
_____ Universal	D. Series of cutting edges

9. The cutting edges of a curet form the:
   A. Back
   B. Face
   C. Tip
   D. Toe

10. The shank of a universal curet is:
    A. Extra rigid
    B. Flexible
    C. Moderately flexible
    D. Rigid

Learning Activities

1. On a typodont, demonstrate wrist motion activation versus digital motion activation. Critique your technique with a student partner.

2. Demonstrate hand pivot and handle roll.

Board Style Review Questions

1. The cutting edge on a sickle scaler is called the:
   A. Cutting edge
   B. Lateral surface
   C. Tip
   D. Toe

2. Which instrument has a more acutely angled shank to facilitate access to the mesial surfaces of posterior teeth?
   A. Gracey 3/4
   B. Gracey 13/14
   C. Gracey 15/16
   D. Gracey 17/18

3. What is the purpose of a knurled handle?
   A. To increase control over the instrument.
   B. Gives the hygienist freedom to position the instrument against the tooth surface as necessary.
   C. Determines the instrument's function.
   D. To prevent musculoskeletal injuries.

4. Identify the instrument that has a longer terminal shank and a shorter blade to enable easier access to distal surfaces of posterior teeth.
   A. Gracey 3/4
   B. Gracey 11/12
   C. Gracey 15/16
   D. Gracey 17/18

5. Simple shanks bend in one plane and are used for posterior teeth. Complex shanks bend in two planes and are used for both anterior and posterior teeth.
   A. Both statements are correct.
   B. The first statement is correct; the second statement is incorrect.
   C. Both statements are incorrect.
   D. The first statement is incorrect; the second statement is correct.

6. All of the following are true of digital motion activation *except* for one. Which one is the *exception?*
   A. Movement of the instrument occurs by flexing three fingers.
   B. This type of activation is recommended for removing calculus.
   C. Can lead to muscle fatigue and repetitive stress injuries.
   D. Less stable than wrist motion activation.

7. A small diameter handle can:
   A. Lessen the hygienist's control over the instrument.
   B. Increase muscle fatigue.
   C. Allow for movement in zones with limited access.
   D. All of the above.

8. Adaptation provides stabilization during instrumentation. It focuses on making the working end of the instrument correspond with the contour of the tooth surface.
   A. Both statements are true.
   B. The first statement is true; the second statement is false.
   C. Both statements are false.
   D. The first statement is false; the second statement is true.

9. All of the following are limitations of a rigid shank *except* for one. Which one is the *exception?*
   A. Tactile conduction
   B. Effectiveness
   C. Pressure
   D. Calculus detection

10. Select the instruments for which digital motion activation should be used.
   1) Explorers
   2) Gracey curets
   3) Periodontal probes
   4) Power instruments
      A. 1 and 3
      B. 2 and 4
      C. 1, 2, and 3
      D. 1, 3, and 4

Active Learning

Refer to the photograph to answer the following questions.

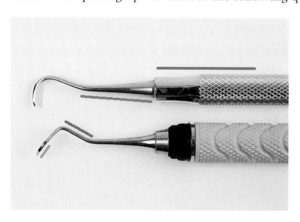

1. Identify the part of the instrument designated by the red line.
   A. Handle
   B. Shank
   C. Terminal shank
   D. Working end

2. Identify the part of the instrument designated by the green line.
   A. Handle
   B. Shank
   C. Terminal shank
   D. Working end

3. Identify the part of the instrument designated by the orange line.
   A. Handle
   B. Shank
   C. Terminal shank
   D. Working end

4. Identify the part of the instrument designated by the yellow line.
   A. Terminal shank
   B. Lateral surface
   C. Point
   D. Toe

REFERENCES

1. Sahayata VN, Patel, VG. Evidence based periodontology. *J Dent Sci*. 2011;2(1):15-19.
2. American Dental Hygienists' Association. Standards for clinical dental hygiene practice. Chicago: American Dental Hygienists' Association. http://www.adha.org/downloads/adha_standards08.pdf. Published March 10, 2008. Accessed June 4, 2012.
3. O'Hehir TE. Debridement = scaling and root-planing plus. *RDH*. 1999;9(5). http://www.rdhmag.com/articles/print/volume-19/issue-5/columns/periodontics/debridement-scaling-and-root-planing-plus.html. Updated 2009. Accessed June 4, 2012.
4. Clerehugh V, Tugnait A, Genco R. *Periodontology at a Glance*. Hong Kong: Wiley-Blackwell; 2009.

Rubrics/Process Evaluations

Process Evaluation Template

Instrument Sharpening: Gracey Curets

Evaluation Criteria	Criteria Met? (Y/N)	Comments
The student...		
Provides rationale for instrument sharpening.		
Selects the appropriate sharpening stone according to the type of dental instrument.		
Establishes a proper angle between the sharpening stone and the cutting edge of the instrument.		
Maintains a constant firm grasp of both sharpening stone and the instrument.		
Ensures that the face of the blade is parallel to the floor.		
Holds the sharpening stone perpendicular to the floor.		
Positions the blade's face at a right angle to the sharpening stone.		
Adjusts the angle of the stone to an obtuse angle of 10° to 20° (Angle of face to stone is 100° to 110°).		
Shifts the instrument toward self to begin sharpening stroke from the shank end to the toe.		
Monitors instrument's contour while sharpening.		
Sharpens the blade's face with a cone-shaped sharpening stone with a slight back and forth stroke (4 to 6 strokes).		
Uses the acrylic stick test to determine sharpness.		
Follows infection control procedures.		

Rubrics/Process Evaluations

Process Evaluation Template

Instrument Sharpening: Universal Curets

Evaluation Criteria	Criteria Met? (Y/N)	Comments
The student...		
Provides rationale for instrument sharpening.		
Selects the appropriate sharpening stone according to the type of dental instrument.		
Establishes a proper angle between the sharpening stone and the cutting edge of the instrument.		
Maintains a constant firm grasp of both sharpening stone and the instrument.		
Ensures that the face of the blade is parallel to the floor.		
Positions the lateral surface of curet so that the angle between the face and stone maintains a 90° value.		
Adjusts the angle of the stone to be more obtuse (10° to 20°). Face to stone is 100° to 110°.		
Shifts the instrument toward self to begin the sharpening stroke from the shank end to the toe.		
Monitors the instrument's contour while sharpening and sharpens around toe to maintain sharp form.		
Uses the acrylic stick test to determine sharpness.		
After surface is sharp, moves to the opposite end and sharpens using the same principles.		
Follows infection control procedures.		

Rubrics/Process Evaluations

Process Evaluation Template		
Instrument Sharpening: Sickle Scalers		
Evaluation Criteria	**Criteria Met? (Y/N)**	**Comments**
The student...		
Provides rationale for instrument sharpening.		
Selects the appropriate sharpening stone according to the type of dental instrument.		
Establishes a proper angle between the sharpening stone and the cutting edge of the instrument.		
Maintains a constant firm grasp of both the sharpening stone and the instrument.		
Ensures that the face of the blade is parallel to the floor.		
Positions the stone in contact with side surfaces of the sickle along its full length.		
Adjusts angle of stone to face (100° to 110°).		
Shifts the instrument toward self to begin the sharpening stroke from the shank end to the toe.		
Uses the acrylic stick test to determine sharpness.		
After surface is sharp, moves to the opposite end and sharpens using the same principles.		
Follows infection control procedures.		

Chapter 27 | Nonsurgical and Surgical Periodontal Therapy

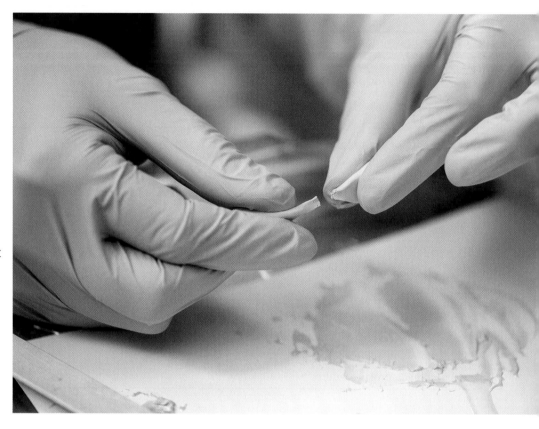

LEARNING OBJECTIVES

After reading this chapter, the student should be able to:

27.1 Explain the goals of nonsurgical and surgical periodontal therapy.

27.2 Outline biofilm formation.

27.3 Demonstrate the use of the perioscope.

27.4 Discuss how periodontal surgery is part of a periodontal rehabilitation protocol.

27.5 Indicate how the dental hygienist supports the periodontal patient in a surgical phase.

27.6 Explain surgical interventions to a patient.

KEY CONCEPTS

• Nonsurgical and surgical therapies may be necessary to control and treat periodontal diseases.

• Periodontal surgery is performed to treat severe periodontal pockets.

• Periodontal surgery follows an appropriate scaling and root planing (SRP) procedure, which is often sufficient to solve the majority of deep pockets.

- Periodontal healing is ideal when periodontal infection is completely eradicated. As a consequence, all surgical procedures have to be considered after periodontal treatment and followed by a dental hygienist.
- It is crucial that dental hygienists be familiar with periodontal surgical and nonsurgical procedures to effectively help their patients in attaining and maintaining periodontal health.

RELEVANCE TO CLINICAL PRACTICE

A number of types of periodontal diseases exist. Untreated periodontal disease can eventually lead to tooth loss and other health problems. Types of periodontal diseases include gingivitis, the mildest and only reversible form, aggressive periodontitis, chronic periodontitis, periodontitis as a manifestation of systemic disease, and necrotizing periodontal disease.[1]

The goal of periodontal therapy is to achieve successful periodontal regeneration. **Scaling and root planing (SRP)**, sometimes referred to as **periodontal debridement**, can solve most periodontal problems, but it is often insufficient when a patient has deep pockets. Regenerative surgery is essential to regenerate a new periodontal apparatus and obtain satisfactory functional and aesthetic results.

Dental hygienists need to be familiar with periodontal surgical and nonsurgical procedures to effectively help their patients attain and maintain periodontal health. If in a general dental practice, and if all treatment measures fail, the patient should be referred to a periodontist. If periodontitis is detected as a manifestation of systemic disease, such as diabetes, the patient should also be referred to a physician.

The Basics

1. How long does it typically take for the junctional epithelium to heal?
   A. 1 week
   B. 2 weeks
   C. 3 weeks
   D. 4 weeks

2. Guided tissue response is:
   A. A procedure attempting to regenerate lost periodontal structures through differential tissue responses.
   B. A definitive procedure designed for the removal of cementum and dentin that is rough and/or permeated by calculus or contaminated with toxins or microorganisms.
   C. A procedure involving the removal of bacterial plaque biofilm and calculus deposits from crown and/or root surfaces and from within the pocket, without root surface removal.

3. Before administering a locally delivered agent, the dental hygienist should provide patient education. In general, what should be discussed with the patient regarding the locally delivered agent?

_____

_____

_____

_____

_____

_____

_____

_____

_____

4. Which restorative surgical procedure is not indicated in cases of active periodontal infection?
   A. Bone graft
   B. Flap surgery
   C. Guided tissue regeneration
   D. Mucogingival surgery

5. Select the best descriptor for lipopolysaccharides (LPS).
   A. Enhance healing by reducing the bacterial load.
   B. Act as endotoxins and elicit a strong immune response in animals.
   C. Have an increased tolerance of microbes within a dense, mature biofilm to antibiotics.
   D. Destroy or inhibit the growth of disease-causing microbes.

6. Which product has doxycycline as an active ingredient?
   A. Arestin
   B. Atridox
   C. PerioChip

7. The active ingredient in PerioChip is:
   A. Chlorhexidine gluconate
   B. Doxycycline
   C. Minocycline
   D. Poly-DL-lactide

8. After nonsurgical periodontal therapy, bacteria repopulate in a specific order. Place the bacteria in order from first (#1) to last (#8) to repopulate.

   _____ Bacteroides

   _____ Capnocytophaga species

   _____ Eusobacterium

   _____ Porphyromonas

   _____ Prevotella

   _____ Spirochetes

   _____ Streptococcus

   _____ Viellonella

9. Identify the locally delivered antimicrobial that when administered alone produces improvements in pocket depth and clinical attachment levels at 9 months that are equivalent to SRP alone.
   A. Arestin
   B. Atridox
   C. PerioChip

10. List the three C's related to clinical response.

1) _____

_____

2) _____

_____

3) _____

_____

Learning Activities

1. Discuss the potential benefits of using lasers for soft tissue procedures.

_____

_____

_____

_____

_____

_____

_____

_____

_____

_____

_____

_____

_____

_____

2. Describe what a healthy periodontal condition should look like clinically.

_____

_____

_____

_____

_____

_____

_____

_____

_____

_____

_____

_____

_____

Board Style Review Questions

1. The greatest period of periodontal healing after nonsurgical therapy occurs between:
   A. 1 to 3 weeks
   B. 3 to 6 weeks
   C. 6 to 12 weeks
   D. 12 to 18 weeks

2. After how many weeks after periodontal therapy should pocket depths be reevaluated?
   A. 1 week
   B. 2 weeks
   C. 3 weeks
   D. 4 weeks

3. Identify the condition for which a gingivectomy is indicated.
   A. To reduce gingival hyperplasia.
   B. When access to the root and bone is desired.
   C. To increase the zone of keratinized gingiva.
   D. To eliminate pockets by positioning the gingival tissue apically.

4. Select the procedure that involves suturing a flap in or near its original position.
   A. Gingivectomy
   B. Osteoplasty
   C. Osteotomy
   D. Replaced flap
   E. Repositioned flap

5. Choose the procedure that relates to the removal of nonsupporting bone to improve bone morphology.
   A. Gingivectomy
   B. Guided tissue regeneration
   C. Osteoplasty
   D. Osteotomy

6. All of the following are predictable outcomes of periodontal healing after nonsurgical periodontal therapy *except* for one. Which one is the *exception?*
   A. New connective tissue attachment to root surfaces.
   B. Periodontal pocket healing.
   C. Resolution of inflammation.
   D. Repair of existing tissues.

7. Choose the factors that can result in reinfection of periodontal pockets.
   1) Residual biofilm
   2) Increased tolerance of microbes
   3) Reservoirs of bacteria in calculus
   4) Reservoirs of bacteria within the dentinal tubules of infected root surfaces and soft tissue.
      A. 1, 2, and 3
      B. 2, 3, and 4
      C. 1, 2, 3, and 4
      D. Only 1

8. After periodontal debridement, the plaque biofilm shifts from predominantly gram-positive flora found in periodontal disease to gram-negative bacteria. There is also an increase in motile forms especially spirochetes after treatment.
   A. Both statements are true.
   B. The first statement is true; the second statement is false.
   C. Both statements are false.
   D. The first statement is false; the second statement is true.

9. Identify the treatment that is believed to facilitate regeneration of lost cementum, periodontal ligament, and the alveolar bone.
   A. Flap surgery
   B. Mucogingival surgery
   C. Osteotomy
   D. Regenerative periodontal surgery

10. The goal(s) for suturing after periodontal procedures is/are:
   1) To provide adequate tension for wound closure.
   2) To reduce postoperative pain.
   3) To permit healing by secondary intention.
   4) To prevent bone exposure.
      A. 1, 2, and 3
      B. 1, 2, and 4
      C. 1, 3, and 4
      D. Only 1

REFERENCES

1. Armitage GC. Development of a classification system for periodontal diseases and conditions. *Ann Periodontol.* 1999;4(1):1-6.

Chapter 28 | Management of Dentin Hypersensitivity

KEY TERMS

Brännström
  hydrodynamic theory
dentin tubules
iontophoresis
myelinated A-delta fiber
smear layer
Tomes fiber

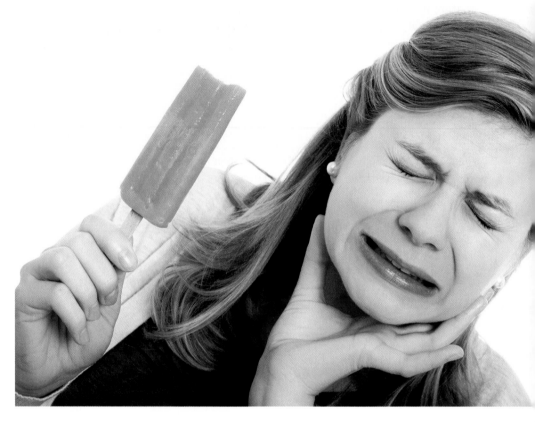

LEARNING OBJECTIVES

After reading this chapter, the student should be able to:

28.1 Describe dentin hypersensitivity and discuss the prevalence, cause, and symptoms.

28.2 Recognize by exclusion the cause associated with various entities of dentin hypersensitivity.

28.3 Identify the most common teeth affected by dentin hypersensitivity and predisposing factors that contribute to this condition.

28.4 Recognize transient and long-term occurrences of dentin hypersensitivity and recommendations for patient relief.

28.5 Discuss and compare preventive and therapeutic modalities in the treatment of dentin hypersensitivity.

28.6 Define the new and widely used generation of medicaments that support prevention and control of symptoms associated with hypersensitivity.

28.7 Develop an evidence-based approach to preventing dentin hypersensitivity in individualized patient cases.

KEY CONCEPTS

- Dentin hypersensitivity has been referred to as one of the most chronic and painful dental conditions that occurs often in the general population but is more prevalent in periodontal patients.
- Differential diagnosis of the cause of dentin hypersensitivity in conjunction with patient education ensures greater success in managing, preventing, and relieving symptoms of hypersensitivity.
- Evidence-based therapies are introducing a new generation of agents that enhance the combination of fluoride with calcium and phosphates in successfully treating chronic and painful symptoms while remineralizing tooth structure.

RELEVANCE TO CLINICAL PRACTICE

Dentin hypersensitivity is a common, chronic, and painful disorder experienced by a majority of the general population. Depending on its frequency and intensity of occurrence, patients may or may not report dentin hypersensitivity during routine dental visits. Dentin hypersensitivity may be transient or persistent and may cause difficulty in normal function on a daily basis.

Dental hygienists should be able to recognize symptoms of dentin hypersensitivity by completing a thorough dental history, examining clinical structures, and applying appropriate treatment modalities that resolve the associated symptoms. With the new diagnostic technologies and therapeutic medicaments available today, the dental hygienist is better equipped to identify and recommend treatment that can minimize or eliminate this dental disorder.

The Basics

1. Arrange the teeth in order from most commonly affected by dentin hypersensitivity to least affected.
   A. Canines, first premolars, incisors, second premolars, molars.
   B. Incisors, canines, first premolars, second premolars, molars.
   C. Canines, incisors, first premolars, second premolars, molars.
   D. First premolars, second premolars, molars, canines, incisors.

2. For the Basic Erosive Wear Examination (BEWE), a score of 2 signifies:
   A. Hard tissue loss greater than 50% of the surface area.
   B. Hard tissue loss greater than 50% of the surface area.
   C. Initial loss of surface texture.
   D. No erosive tooth wear.

3. Select the treatment that decreases tubule diameter and interrupts the nerve transmission and fluid flow to the pulp.
   A. Calcium-phosphate
   B. Glutaraldehyde
   C. Oxalates
   D. Protein precipitants

4. Select the desensitizing agents that are classified as protein precipitants.
   1) Amorphous calcium phosphate
   2) Arginine calcium carbonate
   3) Silver nitrate
   4) Strontium chloride
      A. 1 and 2
      B. 1 and 4
      C. 2 and 3
      D. 3 and 4

5. With regard to sensitivity, the mechanism of action of potassium nitrate is to:
   A. Decrease the permeability of dentin.
   B. Reduce dentin permeability and occlude tubules.
   C. Reduce nerve excitability by blocking repolarization of nerve endings.
   D. Create a precipitate to enable the blocking of open dentinal tubules.

6. Dentin hypersensitivity is described as:
   A. A sharp pain of limited duration that occurs in areas of exposed dentin in response to a stimulus.
   B. A dull pain of unlimited duration that occurs in areas of exposed dentin in response to a stimulus.
   C. A dull pain of limited duration that occurs in areas of exposed dentin in response to a stimulus.
   D. A sharp pain of limited duration that occurs without a stimulus in areas of exposed dentin.

7. All of the following can contribute to dentin hypersensitivity *except* for one. Which one is the *exception?*
   A. Cold air
   B. Osmotic stimuli
   C. Faulty restorations
   D. A fork in contact with exposed surfaces

8. Which class of desensitizing agents occludes dentin tubules and replaces lost minerals?
   A. Calcium phosphate technology
   B. Nerve hyperpolarization agents
   C. Protein precipitants
   D. Tubule obtundants

9. A tubule obtundant should be recommended when:
   A. There is exposed dentin accompanied by symptoms of pain when a thermal stimulus is applied.
   B. There is exposed dentin accompanied by symptoms of pain when a mechanical stimulus is applied.
   C. There is exposed dentin accompanied by symptoms of pain when a chemical stimulus is applied.
   D. There is exposed dentin accompanied by symptoms of pain when any type of stimuli provokes a reaction.

10. After a diagnosis of dentin hypersensitivity, behavioral risks and contributing factors should be identified. List three areas of patient education that the dental hygienist should address.

    1) _____

    2) _____

    3) _____

Learning Activities

1. Explain the hydrodynamic theory. Draw a picture to demonstrate this theory to a patient.

2. Describe the two phases of hypersensitivity development.

_____

_____

_____

_____

_____

_____

_____

_____

_____

_____

_____

_____

_____

_____

_____

_____

_____

_____

_____

_____

_____

_____

_____

_____

Board Style Review Questions

1. Which sensory nerve fibers elicit a well-localized sharp pain considered responsible for dentin hypersensitivity?
   A. Myelinated A-delta fibers
   B. A-beta fibers
   C. C-fibers
   D. Unmyelinated A-fibers

2. To increase its effectiveness, a mild electrical current is applied to a dentifrice, which is applied to the tooth. This process is termed:
   A. Iontophoresis
   B. Laser therapy
   C. Periodontal plastic procedure
   D. Restorative procedures

3. Select the correct mode of action for potassium nitrate.
   A. Calcium phosphate technology
   B. Protein precipitant
   C. Nerve hyperpolarization
   D. Tubule obtundant

4. Choose the best phrase to describe C-fibers.
   A. A well-localized sharp pain.
   B. A sharp pain of short duration; more responsive to electrical stimulation.
   C. A thin layer of organic debris that reduces dentin sensitivity.
   D. Unmyelinated; produce a dull, nonlocalized pain felt from direct pulpal stimulation.

5. For tooth sensitivity, which of these agents provide longer lasting relief?
   A. Adhesives and resins
   B. Calcium compounds
   C. Potassium nitrates
   D. Potassium oxalates

6. The likelihood that a patient will experience dentin hypersensitivity is:
   A. Inversely related to the number of dentin tubules.
   B. Directly proportionate to the number of exposed dentin tubules.
   C. Not related to the number of dentin tubules exposed.
   D. Indirectly related to the type of stimuli applied.

7. Identify the polymerizing agent from these products.
   A. 5% glutaraldehyde
   B. Calcium hydroxide
   C. Fluoride varnish
   D. Glass ionomer cements

8. The result of the basic erosive wear examination (BEWE) is not only a measure of the severity of the condition but also a guide for management. Scores of 1 and 2 indicate dentin involvement.
   A. Both statements are true.
   B. The first statement is true; the second statement is false.
   C. Both statements are false.
   D. The first statement is false; the second statement is true.

9. All of the following are precipitants *except* for one. Which one is the *exception?*
   A. Calcium hydroxide
   B. Calcium-phosphate compounds
   C. Hydroxyethyl methacrylate
   D. Oxalates

10. Which of the following contribute to decreasing dentinal sensitivity?
    1) Professional topical fluoride applications
    2) Home-applied fluoride toothpaste
    3) Formation of reparative or tertiary dentin
        A. 1 and 2
        B. 1 and 3
        C. 1, 2, and 3
        D. Only 1

Chapter 29 | Polishing

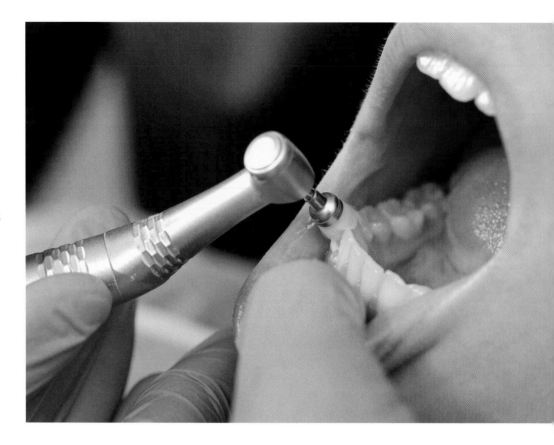

LEARNING OBJECTIVES

After reading this chapter, the student should be able to:

29.1 Explain selective polishing to patients.

29.2 List the indications and contraindications of manual, power, and air polishing.

29.3 Apply the technique of manual, power, or air polishing in the clinical setting.

29.4 Describe the armamentarium needed for each polishing procedure.

29.5 Select a prophy paste or air-polishing powder based on the patients' needs.

KEY CONCEPTS

• Polishing is a technique used to remove extrinsic stain from the enamel surface.

• Evaluating the need for polishing is based on the needs of each patient.

• Selecting the appropriate polishing technique is necessary based on the patient's health history.

RELEVANCE TO CLINICAL PRACTICE

Polishing is a technique that is used on most patients toward the end of a dental hygiene appointment. Different types of polishing methods include manual, power, and air polishing. The purpose of polishing is to remove extrinsic stains that cannot be removed with hand or ultrasonic instruments from enamel surfaces or before sealant placement. Many patients feel the most important part of their hygiene visit is when they have their teeth polished because they "feel smooth and appear shiny and white." It has been suggested that untrained clinicians should not perform polishing because the outer surface of the enamel layer, which contains fluoride, may be removed, and damage to restorative materials including amalgams, composites, and porcelain may occur.[1]

The dentist and dental hygienist are the most qualified clinicians in the dental office to make the decision as to when a patient should receive polishing during an oral prophylaxis appointment.[1] Therefore, learning the types of polishing methods used during a dental hygiene appointment and knowing when to incorporate them is important when assessing a patient. In this chapter, we discuss the different polishing methods, indications, contraindications, and armamentarium used for each procedure.

The Basics

1. Tetracycline causes the enamel to appear:
   A. White-to-brown
   B. Black
   C. Gray
   D. Yellow

2. Selective polishing refers to polishing specific teeth that present with only extrinsic stains. This method is used to reduce potential damage to the enamel, cementum, and dentin.
   A. Both statements are correct.
   B. The first statement is correct; the second statement is incorrect.
   C. Both statements are incorrect.
   D. The first statement is incorrect; the second statement is correct.

3. List and describe the four postprocedure steps for power polishing.

   1) _____
      _____

   2) _____
      _____

   3) _____
      _____

   4) _____
      _____

4. Which of the following does *not* cause intrinsic staining?
   A. Chlorhexidine
   B. Fluorosis
   C. Smoking
   D. Tetracycline
   E. Trauma

5. Extrinsic stain should only be removed by manual, power, or air-polishing techniques. These stains can be caused from smoking, coffee, chorhexidine, and stannous fluoride.
   A. Both statements are correct.
   B. The first statement is correct; the second statement is incorrect.
   C. Both statements are incorrect.
   D. The first statement is incorrect; the second statement is correct.

6. Mohs hardness value for enamel is:
   A. 0.4
   B. 4.0
   C. 5.0
   D. 6.0

7. Air polishing can be used for all of the following conditions *except* for one. Which one is the *exception?*
   A. For heavy extrinsic stain removal
   B. For plaque removal from orthodontic appliances
   C. To remove bacteria in occlusal fissures
   D. To smooth/polish the sealant after placement

8. Explain the purpose of a finishing strip for stain removal and how to use it.

_____

_____

_____

_____

_____

_____

_____

_____

_____

_____

_____

_____

_____

_____

_____

9. Identify the contraindications to air polishing.

1) _____   4) _____

2) _____   5) _____

3) _____   6) _____

Learning Activities

1. Locate and discuss recent research related to the abrasiveness of polishing the enamel surface.

_____

_____

_____

_____

_____

_____

_____

_____

2. Compare and contrast manual polishing to power polishing.

_____

_____

_____

_____

_____

_____

_____

_____

_____

3. What concerns could arise with polishing if it is performed by an untrained clinician?

_____

_____

_____

_____

_____

_____

_____

Board Style Review Questions

1. The purpose of polishing is to:
   1) Remove extrinsic stain
   2) Prepare for sealant placement
   3) Ensure that the teeth feel smooth to the patient
   4) Ensure that they appear clean to the patient
       A. 1 and 2
       B. 1, 2, and 3
       C. 2, 3, and 4
       D. Only 1

2. Stains that can be removed with hand instruments and polishing are called:
   A. Extrinsic stains
   B. Intrinsic stains
   C. Fluorosis
   D. Tetracycline stains

3. Where is black line stain commonly found in the oral cavity?
   A. Maxillary anterior lingual surfaces
   B. Maxillary posterior lingual surfaces
   C. Mandibular anterior lingual surfaces
   D. Mandibular posterior lingual surfaces

4. Which type of stain is commonly seen in children and forms due to poor oral hygiene habits?
   A. Black
   B. Brown
   C. Green
   D. Orange

5. The higher the amount of stain, the more abrasive the paste should be. The more abrasive a prophy paste is, the smaller the grit size.
   A. Both statements are true.
   B. The first statement is true; the second statement is false.
   C. Both statements are false.
   D. The first statement is false; the second statement is true.

6. Which of these ingredients found in prophy paste can be used on enamel and restorations?
   A. Pumice
   B. Glycerin
   C. Glycerol
   D. Feldspar

7. During polishing, which of the following are recommended?
   A. To use a fast speed, heavier pressure, and dry prophy paste.
   B. To use a fast speed, lighter pressure, and dry prophy paste.
   C. To use a slow speed, lighter pressure, and wet prophy paste.
   D. To use a slow speed, heavier pressure, and wet prophy paste.

8. The Mohs hardness value for pumice is:
   A. 0.4
   B. 3.0
   C. 5.0
   D. 6.0

9. The process in which minerals and fluoride are deposited into demineralized areas of the enamel is called:
   A. Desensitization
   B. Remineralization
   C. Hypersensitivity
   D. Therapeutic polishing

10. All of the following ingredients added to prophy paste help to reduce sensitivity or to remineralize the enamel *except* for one. Which one is the *exception?*
    A. Arginine-calcium carbonate
    B. Calcium sodium phosphosilicate
    C. Sodium bicarbonate powder
    D. Fluoride

REFERENCES

1. American Dental Hygienists' Association. Position on the oral prophylaxis. American Dental Hygienists' Association. https://www.adha.org/resources-docs/7115_Prophylaxis_Postion_Paper.pdf. Approved April 29, 1998. Accessed November 24, 2013.

Rubrics/Process Evaluations

Process Evaluation Template		

Air Polishing

Evaluation Criteria	Criteria Met? (Y/N)	Comments
Materials: Student has the necessary items ready before starting the procedure. (All PPE, mirror, air/water syringe, saliva ejector, high-volume evacuator, handpiece, insert, air-polishing powder, floss, gauze, petroleum jelly.)		
Preprocedure. Reviews medical history.		
Student provides patient education.		
Selects appropriate teeth to be air polished.		
Procedure. Preparation: Turns unit on and flushes handpiece with water for 2 minutes.		
Turns the unit off, fills the powder chamber with appropriate air-polishing powder until it reaches the top of the center tube.		
Sets the powder and lavage flow according to amount of stain present (clockwise for heavy stain, counterclockwise for lighter stain).		
Places the insert into the handpiece, turns unit on, and ensures proper flow of water and powder.		
Application. Applies infection control barriers as necessary.		
Uses a modified pen grasp and fulcrum.		
Student aims the insert at the middle third of the tooth, holding the tip 3 to 4 mm away from the surface.		
Student applies a circular motion and avoids aiming the tip at the gingival margin.		
Student polishes 2 to 3 teeth at a time, rinsing frequently.		
Student adapts angle of tip to 60° for anterior teeth, 80° for buccal and lingual surfaces of posterior teeth, and 90° for occlusal surfaces.		
Postprocedure. Evaluation: Ensures that all stain has been properly removed. Flosses to remove powder from interproximal surfaces.		
Uses Standard Precautions during procedure.		
Documentation. Properly documents in patient record.		

Chapter 30 | Esthetics

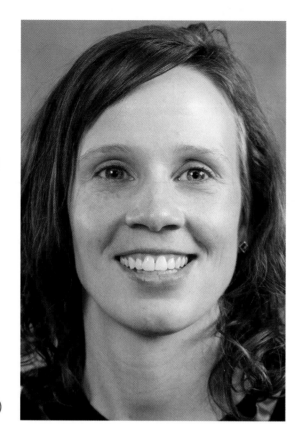

LEARNING OBJECTIVES

After reading this chapter, the student should be able to:

30.1 Discuss various esthetic options to present to the patient.

30.2 Discuss the advantages and disadvantages of esthetic restorations.

30.3 Discuss clinical and homecare techniques of esthetic restorations.

30.4 Explain CAD/CAM technology versus traditional methods of manufacturing.

30.5 Explain the difference between professional and over-the-counter whitening methods.

30.6 Explain mechanism of action, side effects, and contraindications of whitening methods.

30.7 Outline available delivery methods and products for whitening.

30.8 Explain whitening procedures and post-treatment care to the patient.

30.9 Discuss whitening outcomes on various types of enamel.

30.10 Discuss ethical and safety considerations with regard to esthetic dentistry.

30.11 Explain treatment planning considerations for the esthetic patient.

KEY CONCEPTS

• Esthetic dentistry has grown significantly and has changed how dentistry is performed today.

• There are two types of esthetic restorations: direct and indirect.

- CAD/CAM technology has changed the method of fabrication for certain esthetic restorations.
- Dental hygienists play an important role in preserving and maintaining esthetic restorations.
- There are two styles of tooth whitening: professional, which includes in-office and take-home methods, and over the counter.
- Whitening outcomes vary on different types of enamel.
- It is the dental hygienist's role to assist in managing the esthetic patient in all aspects of dental hygiene care, from treatment planning to maintenance.

RELEVANCE TO CLINICAL PRACTICE

Over the past 20 years, the focus on cosmetic dentistry has grown tremendously. Society's belief that a whiter, brighter smile equates with health and physical attractiveness has led to increased interest in elective cosmetic dental procedures. As a result, the use of tooth-colored or esthetic restorative materials and tooth whitening procedures are now very common in today's dental office.

The role of the dental hygienist in presenting esthetic treatment options and maintaining the patient is crucial. The hygienist has the unique opportunity to converse with and treat patients at regular intervals. Thus, the dental hygienist must be well informed about current esthetic treatment options and how they are incorporated in treatment planning, professional maintenance procedures, and patient education.

In this chapter, various esthetic restorative choices are discussed, including composites, crowns, veneers, inlays, and onlays. In addition, a comprehensive review of tooth whitening is presented. This chapter also focuses on dental hygiene considerations for in-office treatment, as well as at-home maintenance of the esthetic patient. Because dental hygienists play a central role in educating and maintaining esthetic patients, hygienists need to be well versed and confident in their knowledge of esthetic dentistry.

The Basics

1. It is difficult to achieve successful whitening results with tetracycline-stained teeth. This type of stain ranges in color from gray, to blue, brown, or yellow. Which colors of stains are more responsive to whitening treatment?
   1) Blue
   2) Brown
   3) Gray
   4) Yellow
       A. 1 and 2
       B. 1 and 3
       C. 2 and 3
       D. 2 and 4
       E. 3 and 4

2. All of the following desensitizing agents can be used in conjunction with whitening treatments *except* for one. Which of these is the *exception?*
   A. Amorphous calcium phosphate
   B. Potassium nitrate
   C. Potassium chloride
   D. Fluoride

3. Compare the following characteristics of indirect and direct restorations.

	Indirect	Direct
Type:	_____	_____
Fabrication:	_____	_____
Cost:	_____	_____
Strength:	_____	_____

4. Professional whitening methods have a much higher concentration of ingredients. The components of professional whitening include both carbamide peroxide and hydrogen peroxide.
   A. Both statements are true.
   B. The first statement is true; the second statement is false.
   C. Both statements are false.
   D. The first statement is false; the second statement is true.

5. List two advantages of a CAD/CAM restoration.

   1) _____

   2) _____

6. Describe the traditional crowning process.

   _____

   _____

   _____

7. Carbamide peroxide breaks down into hydrogen peroxide. A product that contains 20% carbamide peroxide will yield approximately 7% hydrogen peroxide.
   A. Both statements are true.
   B. The first statement is true; the second statement is false.
   C. Both statements are false.
   D. The first statement is false; the second statement is true.

8. Dental hygienists must be able to identify esthetic restorations. List the armamentarium that can be used to aid in determining where restorations exist.

   1) _____   4) _____

   2) _____   5) _____

   3) _____   6) _____

Learning Activities

1. Describe the CAD/CAM process.

   _____

   _____

   _____

   _____

   _____

2. Review the Current Dental Terminology (CDT) codes for veneers. Note the different descriptors between the codes for each type of veneer.

_____

_____

_____

3. Practice using a whitening shade guide on a student partner.

Board Style Review Questions

1. Match the enamel condition terms with the *best* descriptor.

_____ Tobacco stain   A. Brown/yellow staining, white flecks, white spots/striations

_____ Tetracycline stain   B. White spots

_____ Dental fluorosis   C. Brown/yellow staining, blue/gray staining

_____ Hypocalcification   D. Yellowing

2. Select the following phrases that describe an onlay.
   1) Restores the occlusal surface without including the cusps of posterior teeth
   2) Restores the occlusal surface and includes one or more cusps
   3) Direct restoration
   4) Indirect restoration
      A. 1 and 3
      B. 1 and 4
      C. 2 and 3
      D. 2 and 4

3. Select the following phrases that describe an inlay.
   1) Restores the occlusal surface without including the cusps of posterior teeth
   2) Restores the occlusal surface and includes one or more cusps
   3) Direct restoration
   4) Indirect restoration
      A. 1 and 3
      B. 1 and 4
      C. 2 and 3
      D. 2 and 4

4. Glass-ionomer restorations are more commonly used than composites. Glass-ionomer material is fluoride releasing.
   A. Both statements are correct.
   B. The first statement is correct; the second statement is incorrect.
   C. Both statements are incorrect.
   D. The first statement is incorrect; the second statement is correct.

5. All of the following statements are true of a porcelain veneer *except* for one. Which one is the *exception?*
   A. It is prepared outside of the mouth at a dental laboratory.
   B. It is a stronger material than composite.
   C. It is called an indirect veneer.
   D. A porcelain veneer is more polished than a composite veneer.

6. Choose the type of fluoride that is safe for patients with restorations.
   1) Fluoride varnish
   2) Acidulated phosphate fluoride (APF)
   3) Neutral sodium fluoride
      A. 1 and 2
      B. 1 and 3
      C. 2 and 3
      D. Only 1

7. Composite restorations are indirect esthetic restorations. Composite material is a mixture of glass filler particles and polymerizable resin.
   A. Both statements are true.
   B. The first statement is true; the second is false.
   C. Both statements are false.
   D. The first statement is false; the second is true.

8. Which of the following statements is incorrect for composite restorations?
   A. Air-powder polishing is contraindicated.
   B. Ultrasonic devices are contraindicated for use on composite restorations.
   C. Hybrid composites should be polished with medium grit prophy paste.
   D. Hybrid composites should be polished with a water-filled rubber polishing cup.

9. All of the following statements about internal whitening are true *except* for one. Which one is the *exception?*
   A. This procedure is only performed by a dentist.
   B. It involves placing a cotton-soaked pellet of 35% hydrogen peroxide into a pulp chamber.
   C. It is performed on a vital tooth that has suffered trauma resulting in discoloration.
   D. Whitening agents used for internal whitening include carbamide peroxide, hydrogen peroxide, sodium perborate, and calcium peroxide.

10. When educating your patient about the proper care of esthetic restorations, you should recommend that the patient avoid coffee, tea, red wine, and tobacco to prevent staining. Additionally, the patient should be encouraged to use an alcohol-based mouthrinse to reduce plaque retention to the restorations.
    A. Both statements are correct.
    B. The first statement is correct; the second is incorrect.
    C. Both statements are incorrect.
    D. The first statement is incorrect; the second statement is correct.

Rubrics/Process Evaluations

Process Evaluation Template		
Take-Home Professional Whitening (Custom trays)		
Evaluation Criteria	**Criteria Met? (Y/N)**	**Comments**
Student assists the dentist with a comprehensive oral examination.		
Patient is determined a good candidate for take-home professional whitening. Student notes strength of whitening agent prescribed by dentist.		
Patient education provided.		
Informed consent obtained.		
Current tooth shade acquired and documented.		
Intraoral photos taken.		
Risk factors reviewed and explained to patient.		
Acceptable impressions taken.		
Dental stone poured into the impressions to make acceptable models.		
Acceptable plastic trays are made, trimmed, and rough edges smoothed.		
Trays delivered to patient and checked for appropriate fit.		
Demonstration of whitening product insertion into trays.		
Follow-up appointment scheduled.		

Part VII

Anxiety and Pain Management

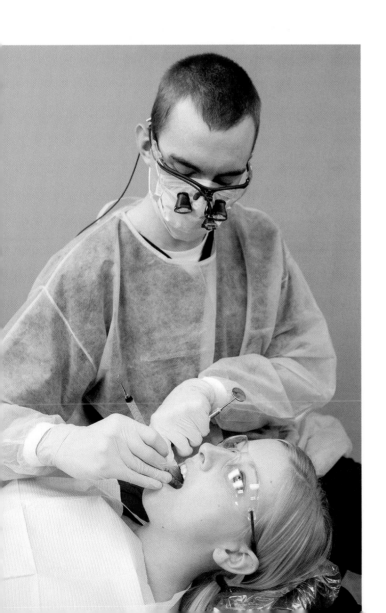

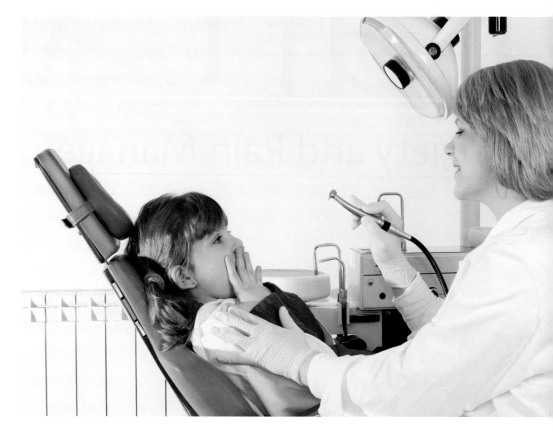

KEY TERMS

dental anxiety
dental fear
dental phobia
iatrosedation
relaxation response
stress response

LEARNING OBJECTIVES

After reading this chapter, the student should be able to:

31.1 Distinguish between dental fear, anxiety, and phobia.
31.2 Identify the causes of dental anxiety and fear, and discuss their effects on patients and the dental team.
31.3 Explain the stress response.
31.4 Assess a patient's degree of fear or anxiety, and plan and implement cognitive and behavioral strategies to reduce dental anxiety and discomfort.
31.5 Apply behavioral strategies to manage anxious children.

KEY CONCEPTS

• Dental fear, dental anxiety, and dental phobia are related, yet distinct.
• Dental fear and anxiety affect people's oral and general health and well-being, lower their pain threshold and pain tolerance, and affect dental hygiene care.
• It is important for the dental hygienist to know the symptoms of the stress response and how to help patients who experience it.
• Establishing a dental fear management program that utilizes assessment tools, communication, and cognitive and behavioral tools is beneficial for patients and clinicians.

- Pharmacological agents provide a role in managing fearful dental patients. Although prescribing and administering them is out of the scope of practice of dental hygienists, they can be part of the dental team's comprehensive dental fear management plan.
- Pain control management is an important aspect of any dental fear management program.
- Managing children who are afraid of dentistry requires different skills than those used for adults.

RELEVANCE TO CLINICAL PRACTICE

Dental fear and dental anxiety are still prevalent among the general population, despite current pain relief measures and dental professionals' awareness of the problem.[1] According to numerous dental fear surveys, between 10% and 20% of adults in the United States avoid seeking regular dental treatment due to extreme dental fear.[2] The prevalence of dental fear has not changed significantly since the 1950s.[2,3] Additionally, various dental fear assessments show that 45% of patients report having moderate dental fear while obtaining oral health care.[4] The problems associated with dental anxiety and fear not only affect the oral health and treatment of a large percentage of the population, but they can also affect the dental clinician's ability to adequately treat his or her patients.[4]

The dental hygienist, being the dental team's prevention specialist and the team member who often spends the most time with patients, has the opportunity to positively affect patients' oral health care by effectively minimizing and managing fear and pain appropriately. Planning and managing patients' dental fears, anxiety, and pain will naturally result in a less stressful work environment for the dental hygienist as well.

The Basics

1. Inviting a younger child to observe an appropriately behaved older sibling have oral health care provided is an example of:
   A. Tell-show-do
   B. Relaxation technique
   C. Modeling
   D. Progressive muscle relaxation

2. All of the following are considerations for using distraction to help reduce a patient's anxiety *except* for one. Which one is the *exception?*
   A. Works best for mildly to moderately anxious patients
   B. Patients may still need a rest break
   C. Works best for longer procedures
   D. May not be effective for patients being administered local anesthesia

3. Match the definition with the appropriate term.

_____ Dental anxiety   A. Significant fear to the degree of being excessive

_____ Dental fear   B. Reaction to a known danger, stimulus, or an immediate threat

_____ Dental phobia   C. Nonspecific ambiguous feeling of unease

4. Select the choice that distinguishes a dental phobic patient from a dentally anxious or fearful patient.
   A. Intensity of the fear of the threat
   B. Immediacy of the threat or stimulus
   C. Anticipation of the threat
   D. Loss of control

5. Identify the cognitive/behavioral technique that is not a relaxation technique.
   A. Focused breathing
   B. Distraction
   C. Guided imagery
   D. Muscle relaxation

6. Select all of the factors that are associated with dental fear and anxiety.
   1) Direct conditioning
   2) Vicarious learning
   3) Personality traits
      A. 1 and 2
      B. 1 and 3
      C. 2 and 3
      D. 1, 2, and 3

7. List three elements that are important when considering how to manage a patient's dental fear and stress response.

   1) _____

   2) _____

   3) _____

8. The verbal interview should include all of the following *except* for one. Which one is the *exception?*
   A. Clinician should demonstrate concern for the patient.
   B. Clinician should portray a calm, confident, reassuring demeanor.
   C. Clinician should provide effective one-way communication.
   D. Clinician should not convey belittlement, criticism, or disbelief.

9. In the presence of fear or anxiety, it can be inferred that pain threshold and pain tolerance:
   A. Increase
   B. Decrease
   C. Stay the same
   D. Are not effected

10. Identify the behavior that the anxious or fearful patient is least likely to exhibit.
    A. Hands gripping the arms of the dental chair
    B. Holding his/her breath
    C. Quiet demeanor, not talking
    D. Hands folded on lap

Learning Activities

1. Explain the benefits of using hypnosis for overcoming dental fear and anxiety.

   _____

   _____

   _____

   _____

   _____

   _____

   _____

   _____

   _____

   _____

2. Describe the "vicious cycle of dental fear."

   _____

   _____

   _____

   _____

   _____

   _____

   _____

   _____

   _____

   _____

3. Review the benefits of a dental anxiety and pain control management program.

   _____

   _____

   _____

   _____

   _____

   _____

   _____

   _____

   _____

Board Style Review Questions

1. For patients who tend to gag, have the patient raise one leg while taking radiographs. This cognitive/behavioral strategy is an example of:
   A. Biofeedback
   B. Desensitization
   C. Distraction
   D. Focused attention

2. All of the following are characteristics of guided imagery *except* for one. Which one is the *exception?*
   A. It is a guided method of relaxation.
   B. It distracts the mind from the outer circumstances.
   C. It uses the imagination of the patient.
   D. It is a natural focused state of mind.

3. The sight of dental instruments can be an immediate threat to a dentally fearful patient. As a result of this threat, the patient may experience bradycardia.
   A. Both statements are true.
   B. The first statement is true; the second statement is false.
   C. Both statements are false.
   D. The first statement is false; the second statement is true.

4. Choose the cognitive/behavioral strategy that is especially useful for teaching patients about new sensations.
   A. Progressive muscle relaxation
   B. Modeling
   C. Tell-show-do
   D. Focused breathing

5. The stress response:
   1) Activates the sympathetic nervous system
   2) Activates the parasympathetic nervous system
   3) Opens blood vessels to allow increased blood flow throughout the body
   4) Constricts blood vessels of the skin
   A. 1 and 3
   B. 1 and 4
   C. 2 and 3
   D. 2 and 4

6. Select the technique in which a patient mentally recites a prayer or phrase (mantra) over and over again.
   A. Focused attention
   B. Modeling
   C. Systemic desensitization
   D. Hypnosis

7. Identify the major difference between dental fear and dental anxiety.
   A. Anticipation of the threat
   B. Loss of control
   C. Immediacy of the threat or stimulus
   D. Stress response

8. Identify the statement that best describes relaxation techniques.
   A. Activation of the parasympathetic nervous system to bring the body back from the fight or flight response.
   B. Tensing and relaxation of individual muscle groups.
   C. Provision of information and a demonstration before proceeding with the procedure.
   D. A natural focused state of mind.

9. Fill in the blank. In the United States, ___ percent of adults avoid seeking dental treatment due to extreme fear.
   A. 0% to 10%
   B. 10% to 20%
   C. 20% to 30%
   D. Greater than 30%

10. Choose the statement that best describes progressive muscle relaxation.
    A. Focuses the mind to assist the body in relaxing the muscles.
    B. Alternating tensing and relaxing the muscles.
    C. Exposes a patient to fearful stimuli while the patient is in a relaxed state.
    D. Focuses the patient on his or her own inner world.

REFERENCES

1. Armfield JM, Stewart JF, Spencer AJ. The vicious cycle of dental fear: exploring the interplay between oral health, service utilization and dental fear. *BioMed Central Ltd*. 2007. doi:10.1186/1472-6831-7-1
2. Heaton L, Carlson C, Smith TA, Baer RA, de Leeuw R. Predicting anxiety during dental treatment using patients' self-reports: less is more. *J Am Dent Assoc*. 2007;138;188-195.
3. Smith TA, Heaton LJ. Fear of dental care: are we making any progress? *J Am Dent Assoc*. 2003; 134(8):1101-1108.
4. Binkley CJ, Gregg RG, Liem EB, Sessler DI. Genetic variations associated with red hair color and fear of dental pain, anxiety regarding dental care and avoidance of dental care. *J Am Dent Assoc*. 2009; 140:896-905.

Chapter 32 | Nitrous Oxide/ Oxygen Sedation

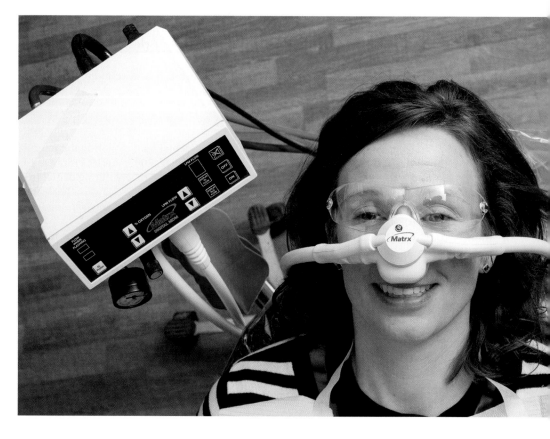

LEARNING OBJECTIVES

After reading this chapter, the student should be able to:

32.1 Explain the advantages and disadvantages of using nitrous oxide/oxygen sedation as compared with other methods.

32.2 Discuss indications and contraindications of the use of nitrous oxide/oxygen sedation.

32.3 Identify the physical, chemical, and pharmacokinetic properties of nitrous oxide and oxygen.

32.4 Discuss the principles of respiration physiology, individual biovariability, and drug titration.

32.5 Recognize the armamentarium used to administer nitrous oxide/oxygen sedation.

32.6 State the importance of informed consent and preoperative patient assessment.

32.7 Describe the appropriation administration technique for nitrous oxide/ oxygen sedation.

32.8 Identify the signs and symptoms of appropriate sedation.

32.9 Describe the procedure for recovery assessment, documentation, and patient dismissal.

32.10 Explain the importance of minimizing nitrous oxide exposure to the operator and office personnel.

32.11 Describe current recommendations for the prudent, ethical, and legal use of nitrous oxide/oxygen sedation for pain and anxiety management.

KEY CONCEPTS

- Nitrous oxide/oxygen sedation is an effective method for managing a patient's pain and anxiety.
- The titration method of administration is the current standard for clinical practice.
- Minimizing exposure to trace gas is important for all members of the health-care team.

RELEVANCE TO CLINICAL PRACTICE

There are many reasons why an individual may need pharmacological assistance during a dental appointment. Unfortunately, patients often present with pain and/or anxiety. Depending on their life circumstances, patients may wait to seek care until their pain is intolerable. And for those with any level of medical/dental anxiety, even the process of seeking care is a traumatic experience. Dental professionals may be called upon to treat both a patient's disease and his or her pain and anxiety. However, professionals have many options to assist these patients. Using nitrous oxide/oxygen sedation appropriately can result in a patient who is relaxed, comfortable, and able to tolerate many types of procedures.

The Basics

1. Why is it important to know your patient's tidal volume?
   A. It determines the amount of flow necessary to maintain patient comfort during respiration.
   B. It determines the level of pain reduction.
   C. It encourages relaxation.
   D. It determines a physiological response.

2. Nitrous oxide is pressurized at:
   A. 650 psi
   B. 700 psi
   C. 750 psi
   D. 2000 psi

3. A nitrous oxide cylinder will be cool to the touch. The amount of gas in the cylinder can be monitored by checking the dial indicator.
   A. Both statements are correct.
   B. The first statement is correct; the second statement is incorrect.
   C. Both statements are incorrect.
   D. The first statement is incorrect; the second statement is correct.

4. Select the phrases that describe appropriate N_2O/O_2 sedation.
   1) The patient's heart rate slows.
   2) Shallow respirations.
   3) Blood pressure decreases.
   4) Patient has control of cough/gag.
      A. 1 and 2
      B. 1 and 3
      C. 1, 2, and 3
      D. 1, 3, and 4

5. After a patient uses nitrous oxide/oxygen sedation, it is advised to administer 100% oxygen postoperatively. For how many minutes should oxygen be administered?
   A. 3 min
   B. 5 min
   C. 7 min
   D. 12 min

6. Nitrous oxide is metabolized in the liver; therefore, patients with hepatitis should not receive nitrous oxide/oxygen sedation.
   A. Both the statement and the reason are correct.
   B. The statement is correct; the reason is incorrect.
   C. Both the statement and the reason are incorrect.
   D. The statement is incorrect; the reason is correct.

7. Which term describes administering a drug in incremental doses over a period of time until a desired endpoint is reached?
   A. Idiosyncratic reaction
   B. Conscious sedation
   C. Anxiolytic
   D. Titration

8. List the advantages of using nitrous oxide/oxygen sedation for a dental appointment.

   1) _____

   2) _____

   3) _____

   4) _____

9. Some machines have floating balls within tubes to show when gas is flowing. How is the actual percentage of nitrous oxide calculated?
   A. By summing the two numbers at the level of both floating balls.
   B. By dividing the N_2O L/min by the total liters per minute.
   C. By subtracting the two numbers at the level of both floating balls.
   D. By multiplying the N_2O L/min by the total liters per minute.

10. Describe the safety features available for nitrous oxide.

    _____

    _____

    _____

    _____

    _____

    _____

    _____

    _____

Learning Activities

1. Repeated exposure to high levels of nitrous oxide whether intentional or unintentional can have a negative biological impact. Discuss protocols that can be implemented to minimize both biohazard risk and personnel exposure.

_____

_____

_____

_____

_____

_____

_____

_____

_____

_____

_____

_____

_____

_____

_____

2. Practice setting up the nitrous oxide/oxygen sedation equipment.

3. Review the rules and regulations in your state for the administration of nitrous oxide/oxygen (N_2O/O_2).

4. Your patient has used nitrous oxide/oxygen sedation to help reduce anxiety during the dental hygiene appointment. Explain to a student partner the process of recovery and assessment for patient dismissal.

_____

_____

_____

_____

_____

_____

_____

_____

_____

_____

_____

_____

_____

_____

Board Style Review Questions

1. During administration of nitrous oxide/oxygen sedation, the reservoir bag should be kept one-third full. If the bag overinflates, there is an excessive and unnecessary amount of gas flow.
   A. Both statements are true.
   B. The first statement is true; the second statement is false.
   C. Both statements are false.
   D. The first statement is false; the second statement is true.

2. The purpose of the flow meter is to:
   A. Mix and adjust nitrous oxide and oxygen.
   B. Prevent gas flow from the wrong line.
   C. Decrease the pressure of the gas from the tank to a level tolerable by human physiology.
   D. Deliver additional gas to the patient if needed.

3. What is the lung capacity of an average adult?
   A. 100 mL
   B. 500 mL
   C. 1000 mL
   D. 1500 mL

4. Which component decreases the pressure of the gas from the tank?
   A. Hose
   B. Nasal hood
   C. Regulator
   D. Reservoir bag

5. The majority of contraindications for use of nitrous oxide/oxygen sedation are relatively uncommon. However, there are situations in which the procedure should be postponed or medical consultation is recommended.
   A. Both statements are correct.
   B. The first statement is correct; the second statement is incorrect.
   C. Both statements are incorrect.
   D. The first statement is incorrect; the second statement is correct.

6. What is the minute volume for the average adult?
   A. 3 to 5 L/min
   B. 6 to 7 L/min
   C. 8 to 10 L/min
   D. 12 L/min

7. All of the following are reasons for oversedation *except* for one. Which one is the *exception?*
   A. The operator administers the drug too quickly.
   B. The dose of the drug is too great.
   C. The drug dose is too fast and too much.
   D. The operator administers the drug in increments.

8. Which of these patients is a candidate for nitrous oxide/oxygen sedation?
   A. Patient who is unable to communicate the drug effects to the dental hygienist.
   B. Patient undergoing cancer treatment with bleomycin sulfate.
   C. Patient diagnosed with bipolar disorder.
   D. Patient diagnosed with hypertension.

9. Nitrous oxide is stored as a liquid in blue cylinders. Nitrous oxide is lighter than air.
   A. Both statements are correct.
   B. The first statement is correct; the second statement is incorrect.
   C. Both statements are incorrect.
   D. The first statement is incorrect; the second statement is correct.

10. Oxygen is pressurized at:
    A. 650 psi
    B. 700 psi
    C. 750 psi
    D. 2000 psi

Rubrics/Process Evaluations

Process Evaluation Template		
Nitrous Oxide/Oxygen Sedation		
Evaluation Criteria	**Criteria Met? (Y/N)**	**Comments**
The student...		
Opens tanks, ensures suction adequacy/ operation, and maximizes ventilation if possible.		
Turns on unit if applicable. Inspects reservoir bag, tubing, and nasal hood. Assembles and connects to unit.		
Assesses medical history, vitals, and purpose for using N_2O/O_2 sedation.		
Acquires informed consent.		
Establishes minute volume.		
Fits nasal hood on patient, securing the strap behind the headrest.		
Fills reservoir bag to 2/3 full if not already filled.		
Adjusts L/min if bag overinflates (decreases O_2) or collapses (add O_2).		
Begins titration by adding approximately 10% to 20% nitrous oxide.		
Waits 1 to 3 minutes before administering additional nitrous oxide in increments of 5% to 10%.		
Monitors signs, symptoms, and patient reaction.		
Does not leave patient unattended.		
Administers a minimum of 5 min of 100% postoperative oxygen.		
Properly documents procedure including patient's tolerance.		
Uses standard precautions during procedure.		
Properly disinfects and sterilizes equipment after patient dismissal.		

Chapter 33 | Local Anesthesia

KEY TERMS

absolute contraindication

acid–base balance (pH)

afferent nerve

amides

depolarize

efferent nerve

ester

infiltration

ischemia

isotonic

local anesthesia

lumen

negative aspiration

nerve block

pharmacokinetics

positive aspiration

relative contraindication

trismus

vasoconstrictor

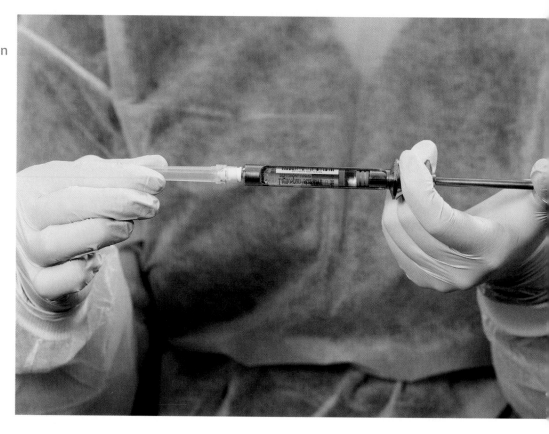

LEARNING OBJECTIVES

After reading this chapter, the student should be able to:

33.1 Articulate the importance of adequate pain control as a prelude to providing quality dental care.

33.2 Describe the physiological mechanism of nerve conduction.

33.3 Explain how local anesthetics prevent nerve transmission.

33.4 Identify and describe the pharmacology of the commonly used local anesthetic agents and vasoconstrictors.

33.5 Recognize disease conditions and medications that may alter or contraindicate the use of local anesthetic agents and/or vasoconstrictors.

33.6 Recognize signs and symptoms of local and systemic complications associated with the administration of local anesthetic agents.

33.7 Explain why local anesthetics may not be as effective in an area of injury (infection).

33.8 Describe the neuroanatomy of the trigeminal nerve.

33.9 Identify the armamentarium for local anesthesia.

33.10 Describe the techniques for administration of local anesthesia.

33.11 Identify the anatomical landmarks associated with administration for the following injections: ASA, MSA, PSA, IO, GP, NP, Gow-Gates and IA nerve block, buccal, mental, and incisive.

33.12 Identify which nerve, teeth, and soft tissue structures are anesthetized with each of the preceding injections.

KEY CONCEPTS

- Local anesthetics play an invaluable role in the provision of the dental hygiene process of care.
- **Local anesthesia** is defined as a temporary loss of sensation in a specific area of the body without loss of consciousness.
- Two major classes of injectable local anesthetics exist: **esters** and **amides.**

RELEVANCE TO CLINICAL PRACTICE

Local anesthetics play an invaluable role in the provision of the dental hygiene process of care. Studies indicate that 10% to 20% of the U.S. population experiences moderate to high levels of dental anxiety. This fear prohibits regular dental visits, resulting in poor oral health.[1] The dental office is unique in that patients often avoid the office because of the fear of pain associated with treatment, yet pain often brings patients to the dental office. Pain is a response that protects the body from harm. Many individuals who are fearful of dentistry worry about receiving oral injections.[2] Patient comfort enables the clinician to provide comprehensive care while reducing anxiety and increasing patient compliance.

The Basics

1. Identify the nerve that innervates the palatal mucosa of the premaxilla area.
   A. Mandibular
   B. Maxillary
   C. Nasopalatine
   D. Ophthalmic

2. The composition of Oraqix is:
   A. 2% lidocaine
   B. 2.5% lidocaine and 2.5% prilocaine
   C. 3% lidocaine
   D. 3% lidocaine and 3% prilocaine

3. Ester-type local anesthetics are likely to cause allergic sensitivities. Amides are metabolized in the plasma.
   A. Both statements are correct.
   B. The first statement is correct; the second statement is incorrect.
   C. Both statements are incorrect.
   D. The first statement is incorrect; the second statement is correct.

4. Consider the administration of local anesthetic for a patient with methemoglobinemia. Which of these statement(s) is/are *incorrect?*
   1) Administration of local anesthetic should be avoided.
   2) Administration of articaine should be avoided.
   3) Administration of lidocaine should be avoided.
   4) Administration of prilocaine should be avoided.
      A. 1
      B. 1 and 3
      C. 2 and 3
      D. 2 and 4

5. The anesthetic in a dental cartridge has a pH of 4.5. This is considered a:
   A. Strong acid
   B. Strong base
   C. Weak acid
   D. Weak base

6. Local anesthesia for the maxillary division of the trigeminal nerve is more successful than for the mandibular division because the maxillary division has fewer variations and is less dense.
   A. Both the statement and the reason are correct.
   B. The statement is correct; the reason is incorrect.
   C. Both the statement and the reason are incorrect.
   D. The statement is incorrect; the reason is correct.

7. You are planning to administer 2% lidocaine HCL with 1:100,000 epinephrine. Determine the maximum recommended dose (MRD) for this patient who weighs 120 lbs.
   A. 3.3 cartridges
   B. 5 cartridges
   C. 5.5 cartridges
   D. 6.7 cartridges

8. What is the duration of Oraquix?
   A. 10 to 20 min
   B. 20 to 30 min
   C. 30 to 60 min
   D. 1 to 1.5 hr

9. Which of these local anesthetics has the longest duration of action?
   A. Carbocaine
   B. Citanest
   C. Septocaine
   D. Xylocaine with epinephrine

10. All of the following contain a vasoconstrictor *except* for one. Which one is the *exception?*
    A. Prilocaine
    B. 2% lidocaine 1:100,000
    C. 3% mepivicaine plain
    D. 4% articaine 1:200,000

Learning Activities

1. Discuss the benefits and risks of vasoconstrictors.

_____

_____

_____

_____

_____

_____

_____

_____

_____

_____

_____

_____

_____

_____

2. Explain how the dental hygienist should address a hematoma that results during an injection.

_____

_____

_____

_____

_____

_____

_____

_____

_____

_____

_____

_____

_____

_____

_____

_____

_____

_____

_____

3. Explain why an area of infection is difficult to anesthetize.

_____

_____

_____

_____

_____

_____

_____

_____

_____

_____

_____

_____

_____

_____

_____

_____

Board Style Review Questions

1. Afferent nerves carry information from the periphery of the body to the peripheral nervous system. Efferent nerve branches carry impulses away from the central nervous system to the periphery of the body.
   A. Both statements are true.
   B. The first statement is true; the second statement is false.
   C. Both statements are false.
   D. The first statement is false; the second statement is true.

2. Which nerve exits the foramen ovale?
   A. Mandibular nerve
   B. Maxillary nerve
   C. Ophthalmic nerve
   D. Trigeminal

3. The process by which the local anesthetic drug is transformed from an active drug to an inactive substance is termed:
   A. Acid-base balance
   B. Depolarization
   C. Metabolism
   D. Pharmacokinetics

4. The mucobuccal fold and the mandibular premolars provide landmarks for which of these injections?
   A. Buccal nerve block
   B. Gow Gates
   C. Inferior alveolar nerve block
   D. Mental nerve block

5. Local anesthetics block the sensation of pain by:
   1) Reducing the passage of Na^+ to depolarize the membrane
   2) Decreasing the amount of Na^+ able to penetrate the cell membrane
   3) Decreasing the permeability of the nerve membrane
   4) Increasing Ca^{++}
      A. 1 and 3
      B. 1 and 4
      C. 2 and 3
      D. 1, 2, and 3

6. Which of these injections is most associated with hematoma formation?
   A. Anterior superior alveolar
   B. Anterior middle superior alveolar
   C. Middle superior alveolar
   D. Posterior superior alveolar

7. The landmarks to consider when administering a greater palatine nerve block include all of the following *except* for one. Which one is the *exception?*
   A. Incisive papilla
   B. Greater palatine foramen
   C. Junction of the maxillary alveolar process and the palatine bone
   D. Maxillary first and second molars

8. Identify the adverse local reaction that can result from needle contact with the medial pterygoid muscle.
   A. Trismus
   B. Hematoma
   C. Paresthesia
   D. Needle breakage

9. A vasoconstrictor causes the lumen of the blood vessel to narrow consequently decreasing blood flow. The systemic effects cause a decrease in blood pressure, heart rate, and oxygen demand.
   A. Both statements are correct.
   B. The first statement is correct; the second statement is incorrect.
   C. Both statements are incorrect.
   D. The first statement is incorrect; the second statement is correct.

10. The greater palatine nerve innervates the:
    A. Buccal mucosa of the molars
    B. Palatal mucosa of the premaxilla area
    C. Posterior soft palate
    D. Posterior lingual gingiva

REFERENCES

1. Prajer R, Grosso G. Quelling the anxiety: Strategies for treating patients with anxiety disorders. *Dim Den Hyg.* 2005;3(6):40-41.
2. Milgrom P, Coldwell SE, Getz T, et al. Four dimensions of fear of dental injections. *J Am Dent Assoc.* 1997;128:756-766.

Rubrics/Process Evaluations

Process Evaluation Template		
Local Anesthetic Administration		
Evaluation Criteria	**Criteria Met? (Y/N)**	**Comments**
The student . . .		
Reviews medical history, investigates potential contraindications.		
Discusses procedure (risks, benefits, alternatives) and acquires informed consent.		
Assembles syringe and tests syringe assembly.		
Wipes the injection site with a clean 2×2 gauze.		
Applies topical anesthetic for 1 to 2 minutes, wipes off excess.		
Retracts lip or cheek for better visibility (holds soft tissue taut between 2 fingers).		
Keeps syringe out of patient's sight.		
Identifies correct area of insertion.		
Inserts needle with bevel to the bone.		
Obtains correct syringe angulation.		
Obtains correct depth of needle penetration.		
Aspirates and proceeds if a negative aspiration is observed or addresses positive aspiration.		
Slowly deposits anesthetic solution (1 to 2 minutes for a full cartridge).		
Observes the patient's reactions, talks patient through procedure.		
Carefully withdraws needle and recaps according to guidelines.		
Properly disposes of needle, syringe, and cartridge.		
Uses standard precautions throughout procedure.		
Properly documents procedure including date, medical status, reason for use, topical and local anesthetic agent used, injection sites, needle type, volume administered, result of aspirations, effect of anesthetic, patient acceptance, any adverse reactions, and instructions provided.		

Part VIII

Evaluation

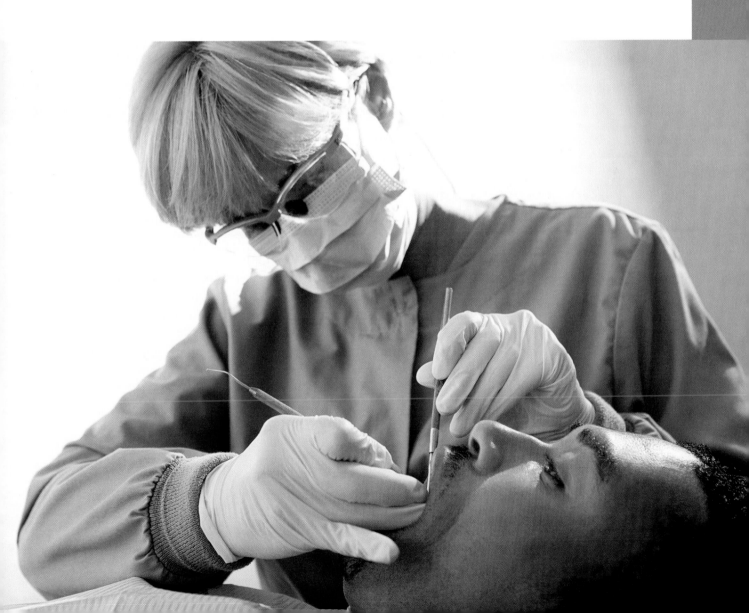

Chapter 34 | Evaluation

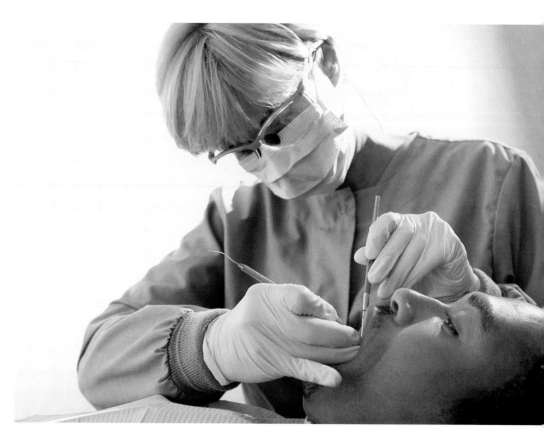

LEARNING OBJECTIVES

After reading this chapter, the student should be able to:

34.1 Describe the taxonomy of the evaluation process.

34.2 Choose the appropriate assessment mechanism to evaluate the outcome of dental hygiene care for all scopes of the practice of dental hygiene.

34.3 Demonstrate the attributes of patient advocacy through effective communication and collaboration with the patient and dental team.

34.4 Formulate an evidence-based, ethical, and legal decision-making process to evaluate the outcome of dental hygiene care in clinical practice and programs.

34.5 Analyze results of treatment implementation to determine prognosis of dental hygiene therapy.

34.6 Recognize the difference between diagnosis and prognosis.

34.7 Identify the criteria for referring a patient to dental specialists.

34.8 Identify the principles of risk management and quality assurance.

KEY CONCEPTS

- Clinical measurements and indices are used for evaluating treatment outcomes.
- Diagnosis determines the disease, and prognosis refers to the prediction for whether or not the patient will heal from that disease.

- Guidelines from dental specialty professions and practice acts provide criteria for referrals to dental specialists.
- Effective communication with patients and other health-care providers is important in evaluation of the dental hygiene process of care.
- Use of evidence-based decision-making assures positive treatment outcomes.

RELEVANCE TO CLINICAL PRACTICE

Mueller-Joseph and Peterson identified evaluation as the fifth phase of the Assessment, Diagnosis, Planning, Implementation, Evaluation, and Documentation (ADPIED) dental hygiene process of care.[1] In 2008, the American Dental Hygienists' Association (ADHA) published the Standards for Clinical Dental Hygiene Practice that recognized the ADPIED as a "critical thinking model of the process of care."[2] Evaluation is the final step in providing comprehensive care for the patient. Subsequently, evaluation is the concluding phase of the clinical reasoning process.

The Basics

1. A formative evaluation involves a description of the soft tissue response to determine the progress of wound healing. A summative evaluation is completed when the odontogram is compared pre- and post-therapy.
   A. Both statements are correct.
   B. The first statement is correct; the second statement is incorrect.
   C. Both statements are incorrect.
   D. The first statement is incorrect; the second statement is correct.

2. Using intraoral photos to compare tissue changes is an example of:
   A. A formative evaluation in the assessment phase of the dental hygiene process of care.
   B. A summative evaluation in the assessment phase of the dental hygiene process of care.
   C. A formative evaluation in the diagnostic phase of the dental hygiene process of care.
   D. A summative evaluation in the diagnostic phase of the dental hygiene process of care.

3. A reliable measurement tool should yield the same results every time. A valid measurement tool measures what it is supposed to measure.
   A. Both statements are correct.
   B. The first statement is correct; the second statement is incorrect.
   C. Both statements are incorrect.
   D. The first statement is incorrect; the second statement is correct.

4. Identify the summative evaluation tools.
   1) O'Leary Plaque Record
   2) CAMBRA
   3) PASS
      A. 1 and 2
      B. 1 and 3
      C. 2 and 3
      D. 1, 2, and 3

5. An example of formative evaluation is:
   A. Comparing vital signs from appointment to appointment
   B. Evaluating the patient's history to determine a diagnosis and plan
   C. Evaluating the extraoral and intraoral tissues
   D. Noting a decrease in blood pressure from the initial appointment to the final appointment

6. The evaluation process is either formative or summative. Formative evaluation is a results process, whereas summative evaluation is an ongoing process.
   A. Both statements are true.
   B. The first statement is true; the second statement is false.
   C. Both statements are false.
   D. The first statement is false; the second statement is true.

7. An example of a summative evaluation is:
   A. Evaluation for caries
   B. Assessing changes in the patient's history
   C. Evaluation of extraoral and intraoral tissues
   D. Clinical evaluation of current studies on diagnosis and therapy to determine the best treatment plan

8. Formative evaluation of the patient's status involves:
   A. Comparing vital signs from the initial appointment to the final appointment.
   B. Taking a biopsy to determine pathology.
   C. Taking and recording patient vital signs at each appointment.
   D. Comparison of the soft tissue response pre- and post-therapy.

9. Identify the type of assessment that the dental hygienist is performing when he/she uses appropriate instruments to achieve maximum tactile sensitivity.
   A. Formative assessment during the implementation phase of the dental hygiene process of care.
   B. Summative assessment during the implementation phase of the dental hygiene process of care.
   C. Formative assessment during the planning phase of the dental hygiene process of care.
   D. Summative assessment during the planning phase of the dental hygiene process of care.

10. When the clinician presents the treatment plan to the patient, he/she can use the patient informed consent (PARQ) process for consent. Define the components of PARQ for patient informed consent.

    P = _____

    A = _____

    R = _____

    Q = _____

Learning Activities

1. How can dental facilities evaluate quality assurance?

    _____

    _____

    _____

    _____

    _____

    _____

    _____

    _____

    _____

    _____

    _____

    _____

2. Outline the three components of the evaluation process according to the ADHA Clinical Standards of Practice.

_____

_____

_____

_____

_____

_____

_____

_____

_____

_____

_____

3. Describe the benefits of using PARQ for obtaining informed consent.

_____

_____

_____

_____

_____

_____

_____

_____

_____

_____

_____

4. Create a list of specialists and contact information to be used for patient referrals.

_____

_____

_____

_____

_____

_____

_____

_____

_____

_____

5. Review referral protocols at your facility.

Board Style Review Questions

1. The orthodontist specializes in treating:
   A. Neuromuscular and skeletal abnormalities.
   B. Diseases and injuries of the pulp and associated periradicular conditions.
   C. Identification and management of diseases affecting the oral and maxillofacial regions.
   D. Research and diagnosis of diseases using clinical, radiographic, microscopic, and biochemical examinations.

2. Your patient has been diagnosed with type 1 diabetes. He/she is most likely under the care of which specialist?
   A. Cardiologist
   B. Endocrinologist
   C. Endodontist
   D. Oral maxillofacial pathologist

3. The role of the clinician in summative evaluation during the assessment phase of the dental hygiene process of care is to:
   A. Obtain informed consent.
   B. Use the evidence-based decision-making process.
   C. Document and communicate expected and real outcomes.
   D. Evaluate histories at each appointment.

4. The O'Leary Plaque Record can be used to:
   A. Discern normal and abnormal tissues.
   B. Screen for potential pathology.
   C. Compare tissue response pre- and post-therapy.
   D. Determine a self-care regimen.

5. Which human need is addressed when the dental hygienist educates the patient and allows him/her to make decisions about their own health?
   A. Conceptualization and problem solving
   B. Protections from health risks
   C. Responsibility for oral health
   D. Wholesome facial image

6. Which of the following are measurable outcomes of dental hygiene care?
   1) Bleeding points
   2) Plaque control
   3) Probing
   4) Retention of sealants
      A. 1 and 2
      B. 1, 2, and 3
      C. 2 and 3
      D. 1, 2, 3, and 4

7. A patient presents for scaling and root planing. He reports a fractured tooth and states that he is not having any pain. The clinician should not proceed with scaling and root planing, because restorative therapy should be completed first.
   A. Both the statement and the reason are correct.
   B. The statement is correct; the reason is incorrect.
   C. Both the statement and the reason are incorrect.
   D. The statement is incorrect; the reason is correct.

8. How can the human need of a wholesome facial image be met?
   A. The clinician provides comprehensive care.
   B. The clinician provides recommendations to improve function and esthetics.
   C. The clinician provides pain management.
   D. The clinician provides caries preventive strategies.

9. How can the human need for a biologically sound dentition be met?
   A. The clinician provides comprehensive care.
   B. The clinician provides recommendations to improve function and esthetics.
   C. The clinician provides pain management.
   D. The clinician provides caries preventive strategies.

REFERENCES

1. Mueller-Joseph L, Peterson M. *Dental hygiene process: diagnosis and care planning.* Albany, NY: Delmar; 1995. 178 p.
2. American Dental Hygienists' Association. Standards for clinical dental hygiene practice. *Access.* 2008;5(3):3-15.

Chapter 35 | Maintenance

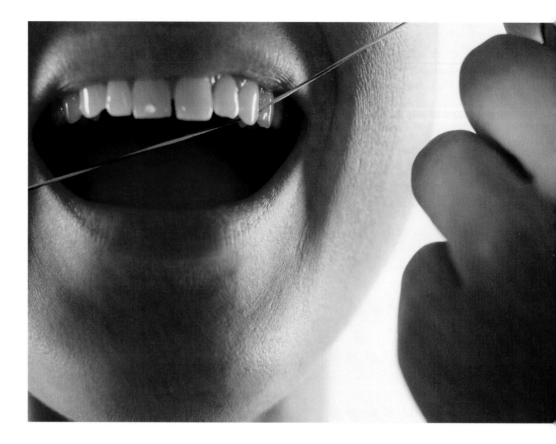

LEARNING OBJECTIVES

After reading this chapter, the student should be able to:

35.1 Evaluate the roles of the dental hygienist, dental team, and patient in maintaining dentition.

35.2 Relate concepts of evaluation to the maintenance phase of dental hygiene therapy.

35.3 Identify contributing factors and signs of the recurrence of dental diseases.

35.4 Make evidence-based decisions regarding medicaments and adjunct treatments for patients in the maintenance phase.

KEY CONCEPTS

- Determine the criteria for a maintenance care plan, including proper continuing care intervals based on the patients' risk assessment.
- Oral maintenance is an important part of overall health.
- Dental implants, when present, are an important part of the maintenance care plan and may require therapy adjustments.
- The maintenance appointment may include locally delivered antimicrobials, depending on the patient's oral risk assessment and periodontal findings.

RELEVANCE TO CLINICAL PRACTICE

Oral health maintenance is an important part of the dental hygiene treatment plan. It is the means for the patient to maintain healthy tissue and dentition free of disease. The hygienist is the preventive specialist in the dental practice. **Maintenance** is an ongoing treatment that occurs either after active therapy or as a routine prophylaxis. The hygienist collects assessment data, provides a dental hygiene diagnosis based on assessment data, implements appropriate therapy, evaluates treatment outcomes, and documents outcomes of therapy.

The Basics

1. Explain how the dental hygienist can help the patient increase self-efficacy through behavior modification.

_____

_____

_____

_____

_____

_____

_____

_____

_____

2. A patient with severe chronic periodontitis should be:
   A. Managed by the dentist and the dental hygienist.
   B. Managed by the dentist.
   C. Comanaged by the referring dentist and periodontist.
   D. Treated by the periodontist.

3. The prognosis for patients who maintain a regular periodontal maintenance schedule is better than for patients who are irregular about their care. The number of teeth lost by noncompliant patients is approximately five times greater than for patients who are compliant.
   A. Both statements are correct.
   B. The first statement is correct; the second statement is incorrect.
   C. Both statements are incorrect.
   D. The first statement is incorrect; the second statement is correct.

4. Select the appropriate guideline(s) for when to use locally delivered antimicrobials.
   1) There is bleeding on probing without any systemic medication effects.
   2) An implant is showing signs of failure.
   3) The pockets must be ≥4 mm.
      A. 1 and 2
      B. 1 and 3
      C. 2 and 3
      D. Only 1

5. Identify the nonmodifiable risk factor for periodontal disease.
   A. Aging
   B. Patient compliance
   C. Smoking
   D. Type 2 diabetes

6. Which criteria must the dental hygienist use to determine a maintenance care plan?
   A. Risk factors
   B. Medical status
   C. Assessment data
   D. Outcomes

7. All of the following medications are contraindicated for pregnant patients *except* for one. Which one is the *exception?*
   A. Arestin
   B. Atridox
   C. Minocycline hydrochloride
   D. PerioChip

8. The chlorhexidine chip is contraindicated for:
   A. Pregnant patients
   B. Pockets less than 5 mm
   C. Patients with developing teeth
   D. Patients with an allergy to minocycline or doxycycline

9. Identify the medication that when combined with scaling and root planing (SRP) produces better outcomes for patients with diabetes compared with SRP alone.
   A. Chlorhexidine
   B. Doxycycline
   C. Minocycline Hydrochloride
   D. PerioChip

10. List the components of assessment that are considered standard protocol for a periodontal maintenance appointment.

   1) _____   5) _____

   2) _____   6) _____

   3) _____   7) _____

   4) _____   8) _____

Learning Activities

1. Group Discussion. In a group of two to three students, review and discuss the recommendations for referral to a periodontist (Box 35-1 in your textbook).

2. Explain how the dental hygienist can detect signs of recurrence of dental disease.

   _____

   _____

   _____

   _____

   _____

   _____

   _____

   _____

Board Style Review Questions

1. While caring for adult patients, vital signs must be taken during the dental hygiene appointment. The hygienist may be one of the first health-care providers to identify a medical concern through the recording of vital signs.
   A. Both statements are true.
   B. The first statement is true; the second statement is false.
   C. Both statements are false.
   D. The first statement is false; the second statement is true.

2. Bitewing radiographs are used to:
   1) Detect caries
   2) Monitor bone levels and assess the quality of interproximal bone
   3) Determine furcation involvement
   4) Detect calculus deposits
      A. 1 and 2
      B. 1, 2, and 3
      C. 1, 2, 3, and 4
      D. Only 1

3. For the patient who is smoking, the dental hygienist can expect all of the following *except* for one. Which one is the *exception?*
   A. More bleeding
   B. More calculus
   C. Greater attachment loss
   D. Deeper pockets

4. Smoking is one of the most significant risk factors for periodontal disease. The patient who quits using tobacco still has an increased risk of attachment loss compared with the patient who has never smoked.
   A. Both statements are correct.
   B. The first statement is correct; the second statement is incorrect.
   C. Both statements are incorrect.
   D. The first statement is incorrect; the second statement is correct.

5. Which of these is not considered a risk factor for a patient with diabetes?
   A. Gingival hyperplasia
   B. Aggressive periodontitis
   C. Periodontal abscess
   D. Calculus deposits

6. Informed consent must be discussed and signed by the end of the appointment. It should include the reason for treatment, risks/benefits, risks of not accepting treatment, time to ask questions, and adequate time to accept/decline treatment.
   A. Both statements are true.
   B. The first statement is true; the second statement is false.
   C. Both statements are false.
   D. The first statement is false; the second statement is true.

7. Periodontal maintenance is:
   1) Care that is provided to the patient with no disease present.
   2) Care that is provided to the patient who exhibits localized areas of active disease.
   3) Therapy that goes beyond prophylaxis because of the provision of site-specific scaling and root planing in areas that have shown disease progression.
   4) The removal of plaque, stain, and calculus.
      A. 2 and 3
      B. 2, 3, and 4
      C. Only 1
      D. Only 3

8. Select the best phrase to complete the following statement. The dental hygiene diagnosis does not focus just on the disease state but also on the:
   A. Risk assessment
   B. Patient's home care
   C. Reason for the problem
   D. Major etiologic factor in periodontal disease

9. What does the A1C measure?
   A. Cardiac enzyme level
   B. Blood clotting factor within the last 12 weeks
   C. Glucose levels within the last 12 weeks
   D. Blood cholesterol level

10. For how many days is minocycline effective?
    A. 7
    B. 7 to 10
    C. 21
    D. 28 to 30

Part IX

Caring for Patients with Special Needs

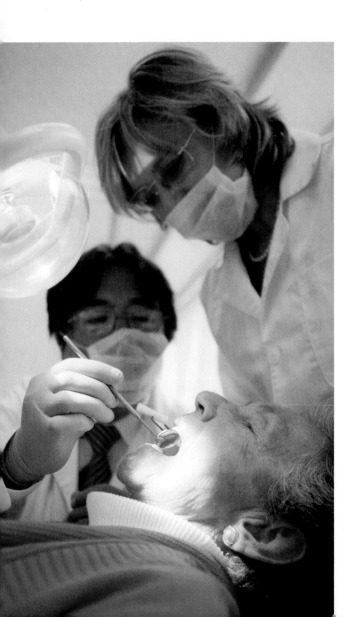

Chapter 36 | Introduction to Special Needs

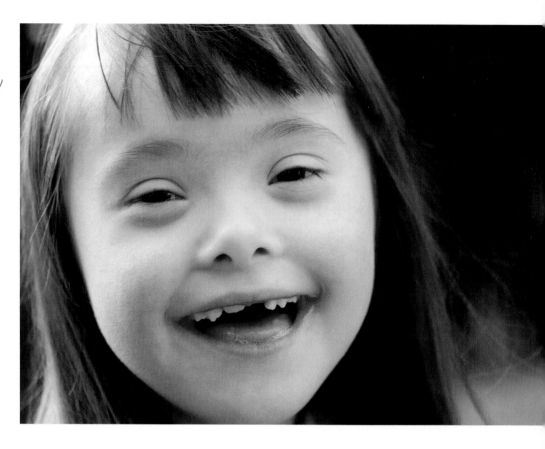

LEARNING OBJECTIVES

After reading this chapter, the student should be able to:

36.1 Identify terms appropriate for patients with special needs.

36.2 Manage patients with developmental disabilities or complex medical issues.

36.3 Describe best practices to interact with patients with special health-care needs.

36.4 Implement a strategy for determining an individualized treatment approach for patients with special needs.

KEY CONCEPTS

• Categorizing patients appropriately based on their developmental disabilities will help the clinician recognize best practices in formulating treatment plans.

• Having a clear understanding of behavioral and medical management allows the clinician to acknowledge that traditional methods of practice may not appropriate for the needs of patients with developmental disabilities.

• Understanding dental interventions that are suitable for patients with developmental disabilities aids in easier transition for the dental team.

RELEVANCE TO CLINICAL PRACTICE

It has been established that people with complex medical and developmental conditions experience more oral health problems than those who do not have these conditions.[1] Advances in medicine have increased the life expectancy of patients with complex medical and developmental disabilities. Thirty years ago, a person with Down syndrome had a life expectancy of about 12 years, compared with 60 years today.[1] For those with special health needs, dental care has been shown to be the number one unmet health-care priority. The many challenges of service delivery to this patient population include patient dexterity, patient cooperation, dependency on other care providers, and lack of available dental care facilities and access to care. Many offices and dental team members have not had adequate experiences in their dental education and elect not to treat this underserved population. As a result, increasing numbers of patients with complex medical and developmental conditions are seeking oral health-care providers with the appropriate knowledge, skills, and abilities to manage their treatment.[2]

The Basics

1. Fill in the table with the treatment considerations for each of the listed conditions.

Condition	Treatment Considerations
Cardiovascular fitness	
Respiratory tolerance	
Neurological concerns	
Hepatic (liver) function	
Renal (kidney) function	

2. Your patient has received local anesthesia during the dental appointment. Which of these is a vasodilator that can be used to reverse the feeling of numbness in soft tissue at the end of the appointment?
   A. Epinephrine
   B. Levonordefrin
   C. Norepinephrine
   D. Phentolamine mesylate

3. What visual cues should the dental hygienist notice when assessing caries risk for a patient with special needs?

   _____   _____

   _____   _____

   _____   _____

4. Using picture boards to familiarize the patient with office procedures is an example of:
   A. Desensitization
   B. Partnership
   C. Time management
   D. Visualization

5. Which of these "best practices" is *most* appropriate for decreasing the stress of a new situation or appointment for a patient with special needs?
   A. Consider having the patient take a mood altering medication.
   B. Use the tell-show-do method.
   C. A friend or family member accompanies the patient.
   D. Use a restriction device as it provides feelings of security.

6. Self-care disability is defined as:

   _____

   _____

7. What is the first step in providing care for patients with complex medical or developmental conditions?

   _____

   _____

8. Choose the category of disability that defines behaviors associated with inappropriate social interrelations.
   A. Cognitive disability
   B. Sensory disability
   C. Self-care disability
   D. Psychosocial disability

Learning Activities

1. Using Table 36-3 from the textbook, discuss how decisions can be made regarding the ability to treat a patient with special needs in the clinical office setting.

   _____

   _____

   _____

   _____

2. Discuss modifications that the dental hygienist can make to oral hygiene products for a patient who lacks dexterity or strength.

   _____

   _____

   _____

Board Style Review Questions

1. The caregiver is essential to consistency and patient management. All of the following are correct statements related to caregiver involvement *except for* one. Which one is the *exception?*
   A. The caregiver is the legal guardian and should provide consent for treatment.
   B. The caregiver has usually not received formal training on how to provide oral care for the patient.
   C. The caregiver can provide information regarding the patient's likes and dislikes.
   D. The caregiver can help determine the best approach for a task.

2. Choose the term that defines multiple chronic diseases.
   A. Psychosocial disabilities
   B. Developmental disabilities
   C. Special needs
   D. Comorbidities

3. The dental operatory must accommodate patients with wheelchairs and walkers. This is mandated by the:
   A. American Dental Association (ADA)
   B. American Association of People with Disabilities (AAPD)
   C. Americans with Disabilities Act (ADA)
   D. Disability Resource Association

4. The dental hygienist should allow the patient to become familiar with equipment and materials. This process is called:
   A. Desensitization
   B. Partnership
   C. Stabilization
   D. Visualization

5. Identify the phrase that best represents people-first language.
   A. The patient is diabetic.
   B. The patient with a hearing impairment.
   C. The patient is hypertensive.
   D. The patient has cardiac disease.

6. Timing of the dental hygiene appointment can affect the outcome of the appointment. For many patients, afternoon appointments are best to ensure that the patient is ready for a new experience.
   A. Both statements are correct.
   B. The first statement is correct; the second statement is incorrect.
   C. Both statements are incorrect.
   D. The first statement is incorrect; the second statement is correct.

7. Select the best definition for dental patients with special needs.
   A. Patients with physical impairment that make it necessary to modify normal dental routines in order to provide dental treatment for that individual.
   B. Patients with medical, psychological, or physical impairments that make it necessary to modify normal dental routines in order to provide dental treatment for that individual.
   C. Patients with medical, physical, psychological, or social situations that make it necessary to modify normal dental routines in order to provide dental treatment for that individual.
   D. Patients with mental and physical impairments that make it necessary to modify normal dental routines in order to provided dental treatment for that individual.

8. What is the purpose of an anxiolytic drug?
   A. To treat diabetes.
   B. To treat cognitive impairments.
   C. To treat hyposalivary function.
   D. To treat anxiety.

9. How can a trusting relationship be established with a patient who is anxious?
   A. The clinician can learn about past experiences.
   B. The clinician can determine the patient's level of understanding.
   C. The clinician can adjust the time interval between appointments.
   D. The clinician can ask questions in multiple ways.

10. Why do most individuals fear dentistry?
   A. They are hypersensitive.
   B. They must give up control of their environment for a period of time.
   C. They are in a new situation.
   D. They have experienced a traumatic event.

REFERENCES

1. Glassman P, Subar P. Planning dental treatment for people with special needs. *Dent Clin N Am.* 2009;53(2):195-205.
2. Glassman P, Subar, P. Creating and maintaining oral health for dependent people in institutional settings. *J Pub Health Dent.* 2010;70:540-548.

Chapter 37 | Cardiovascular Disease

KEY TERMS

angina pectoris
anticoagulant therapy
arrhythmias
atheroma
atherosclerosis
atrial septal defect
bacteremia
bradycardia
cardiovascular surgery
congenital heart disease
coronary heart disease
cytokines
heart block
heart failure
hypertension
infective endocarditis
inflammation
ischemic heart disease
myocardial infarction
patent ductus arteriosus
periodontal disease
post–cardiovascular
  surgery
regurgitation
rheumatic heart disease
stenosis
tachycardia
thrombogenic
thrombus
ventricular fibrillation
ventricular septal defect
ventricular tachycardia

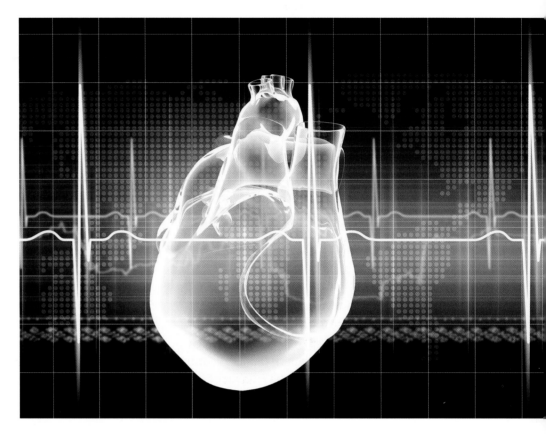

LEARNING OBJECTIVES

After reading this chapter, the student will be able to:

37.1 Identify cardiovascular diseases most commonly encountered in dental hygiene practice.

37.2 Explain the role of inflammation developed in response to the bacterial action in plaque and its link with cardiovascular disease.

37.3 Develop individualized dental hygiene care plans for patients with cardiovascular disease.

37.4 Implement the necessary dental hygiene treatment modifications for patients with various cardiovascular conditions.

KEY CONCEPTS

- Cardiovascular disease (CVD) is a leading cause of death in the United States.
- Dental hygienists must be aware of their patients' general health and recognize the signs and symptoms of CVD.
- Dental hygienists must be able to identify the cardiovascular conditions that prohibit or delay dental treatment, and assess, manage, and treat individuals with controlled cardiovascular disease.

- The assessment and treatment of the patient with CVD require an interdisciplinary approach by the dental hygienist, the dentist, and the patient's physician(s).
- Some of the risk factors associated with CVD are also identified as risk factors for periodontal disease.
- Chronic inflammation and tissue damage, which can result from periodontal disease, give bacteria an opportunity to disseminate to other organs and initiate infections in the host, including cardiovascular disease.
- Evidence-based studies are currently being conducted to determine whether the relationship between periodontal infections and CVD is a direct or an indirect relationship.
- Oral health can have profound consequences for cardiovascular health.
- An accurate medical history and knowledge of the patient's medications can assist the dental hygienist in recognizing and determining whether a patient has CVD.
- To help determine the type of CVD the patient suffers from, the dental hygienist should ask specific questions relative to the patient's medications.
- Dental hygiene treatment modifications should be made specifically to address the patient's type of CVD, medications, and symptoms experienced during treatment.
- Depending on the type of CVD and the patient's symptoms, dental hygiene treatment modifications for patients with CVD include measuring blood pressure before initiation of treatment and during treatment, minimizing the patient's stress and anxiety, careful consideration and use of local anesthesia, placing the patient in a reclined position rather than in a supine position, consulting the patient's physician before initiating treatment, and not treating the patient at this time.
- It is crucial for the dental hygienist to develop individualized oral health-care instructions and recommendations for patients with cardiovascular disease.
- Effective oral hygiene homecare is essential for patients with cardiovascular disease.

RELEVANCE TO CLINICAL PRACTICE

Due to increased life expectancy, dental hygienists are encountering and treating patients with a myriad of health disorders that not only affect their dental health, but also have profound effects on their dental treatment. Among the disorders that may be encountered is cardiovascular disease (CVD). According to the Centers for Disease Control and Prevention, cardiovascular disease is the leading cause of death in the United States for both men and women.[1] CVD encompasses many conditions, such as hypertension, heart failure, angina, infective bacterial endocarditis, valvular defects, and coronary heart disease. As a consequence of this, hygienists are more frequently encountering patients with implantable cardio-defibrillators and pacemakers, and patients with history of **cardiovascular surgery**. Moreover, multiple studies have shown a link between CVD and **periodontal**

disease. Therefore, it is important that dental hygienists recognize the signs and symptoms of CVD, identify the cardiovascular conditions that prohibit dental treatment, and assess, manage, and treat individuals with controlled cardiovascular disease. Due to the risk factors associated with CVD, the assessment and treatment of individuals with CVD requires an interdisciplinary approach by the dental hygienist, the dentist, and the patient's physician(s).

This chapter addresses the association between oral and systemic health and the following cardiovascular diseases:

- Arrhythmias
- Atherosclerosis
- Congenital heart disease
- Heart failure
- Hypertension
- Infective endocarditis
- Ischemic heart disease
  - Angina pectoris
  - Myocardial infarction
  - Chronic ischemic heart disease
  - Sudden cardiac death
- Post–cardiovascular surgery
- Rheumatic heart disease

Suggestions for treatment modifications and dental hygiene considerations and precautions during treatment provided to these individuals are addressed, as is the link between CVD and periodontal disease.

The Basics

1. Identify the strongest chamber of the heart.
   A. Left atrium
   B. Right atrium
   C. Left ventricle
   D. Right ventricle

2. Your patient presents with a blood pressure value of 139/90 mm Hg. Classify this assessment.
   A. Normal
   B. Prehypertension
   C. Stage 1 hypertension
   D. Stage 2 hypertension

3. Identify the term that describes valvular heart disease that occurs when the left ventricle pumps blood to the aorta and the mitral valve falls backward into the left atrium.
   A. Aortic regurgitation
   B. Aortic stenosis
   C. Mitral valve regurgitation
   D. Mitral valve prolapse

4. A normal range for an International Normalized Ratio (INR) value is:
   A. 0 to 1
   B. 1 to 2
   C. 2 to 3
   D. Greater than 3

5. Which type of heart disease occurs commonly in the elderly as a result of atherosclerosis?
   A. Patent ductus arteriosus
   B. Ventricular septal defect
   C. Atrial septal defect
   D. Chronic ischemic

6. Identify the correct dental hygiene treatment modification for a patient with known heart failure.
   A. Patients who are monitored closely by their physicians do not require any treatment modifications.
   B. The patient should be called the day before treatment to remind him/her to bring the latest prothrombin time (PT) blood test to the appointment.
   C. The patient should be called the day before treatment to remind him/her to bring their nitroglycerin to the appointment.
   D. Antibiotic premedication should be considered before dental treatment.

7. Periodontal infections can stimulate:
   1) Fibrinogen production
   2) C-reactive protein production
   3) Platelet aggregation
      A. 1 and 2
      B. 1 and 3
      C. 2 and 3
      D. 1, 2, and 3

8. Select the degree of heart block experienced by a patient who has an absence of conduction between the sinoatrial node and the ventricles.
   A. First degree
   B. Second degree
   C. Third degree
   D. Fourth degree

9. Select the normal range for PT.
   A. 0 to 6 sec
   B. 6 to 10 sec
   C. 10 to 12 sec
   D. 12 to 15 sec

10. Explain how to manage a patient with symptoms of myocardial infarction (MI).

   _____

   _____

   _____

Learning Activities

1. Discuss the prevalence and incidence of hypertension.

   _____

   _____

   _____

   _____

2. Examine the dental hygiene considerations for a patient who is receiving anticoagulant therapy other than aspirin

_____

_____

_____

_____

3. Review the American Dental Association (ADA) recommendations for premedication for patients post-cardiovascular surgery.

_____

_____

_____

_____

Board Style Review Questions

1. All of the following are correct of cardiac arrhythmias *except* for one. Which one is the *exception?*
   A. Result of impulse formation and/or impulse conduction error
   B. Cause abnormal heart rhythms
   C. Can result in tachycardia or bradycardia
   D. Occur only in diseased hearts

2. A sinus node dysfunction that results in less than 60 beats per minute is defined as:
   A. Arrhythmia
   B. Atheroma
   C. Bradycardia
   D. Tachycardia

3. Ventricular tachycardia (VT) is:
   A. Three or more consecutive depolarizations occurring at more than 100 beats per minute.
   B. A skipped heartbeat, a strong beat, or a feeling of suction in the chest.
   C. Uncoordinated contraction of the ventricle cardiac muscle.
   D. Malfunction of the heart's electrical system.

4. A blood pressure value of 130 mm Hg over 85 mm Hg is classified as:
   A. Normal
   B. Prehypertension
   C. Stage 1 hypertension
   D. Stage 2 hypertension

5. Choose all of the following that apply to acute infective endocarditis.
   1) Requires treatment with IV antibiotics
   2) Most often caused by *S. aureus*
   3) Most often caused by *viridians streptococci*
   4) Onset occurs over a period of 6 months
      A. 1 and 2
      B. 2 and 3
      C. 1, 2, and 3
      D. 1, 2, and 4

6. Choose the term that best describes insufficient blood flow to the heart.
   A. Angina pectoris
   B. Congenital heart disease
   C. Ischemic heart disease
   D. Rheumatic heart disease

7. Select all of the phrases that apply to atherosclerosis.
   1) A buildup of fibro-fatty deposit or plaque on the walls of arteries.
   2) Causes a narrowing of the lumen of the vessel.
   3) The main cause of angina pectoris.
   4) A type of arrhythmia.
      A. 1, 2, and 3
      B. 2 and 3
      C. 2, 3, and 4
      D. Only 4

8. Tachycardia refers to a heart rate that is abnormally high. A fast heart rate is of greater concern than a slow heart rate.
   A. Both statements are true.
   B. The first statement is true; the second is false.
   C. Both statements are false.
   D. The first statement is false; the second statement is true.

9. Choose the statement that best defines premature ventricular contractions (PVC).
   A. Three or more consecutive depolarizations occurring at more than 100 beats per minute.
   B. A skipped heartbeat, a strong beat, or a feeling of suction in the chest.
   C. Uncoordinated contraction of the ventricle cardiac muscle.
   D. Malfunction of the heart's electrical system.

10. If a patient presents with stage 2 hypertension, the dental hygienist should:
    A. Allow the patient a few minutes to relax before starting treatment.
    B. Proceed with treatment but monitor blood pressure throughout the appointment.
    C. Refer the patient directly to his/her physician/emergency room.
    D. Evaluate the risk and benefits of using local anesthesia with a vasoconstrictor.

REFERENCES

1. Murphy SL, Xu J, Kochanek, KD, Centers for Disease Control and Prevention. Deaths: preliminary data for 2010. *National Vital Statistics Reports*. 2010;60(4):1-69.

Chapter 38 | Respiratory

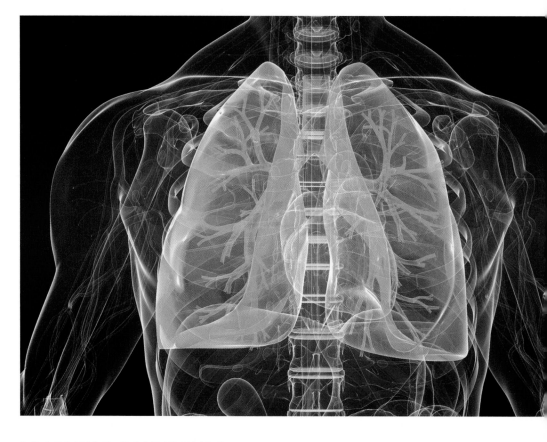

LEARNING OBJECTIVES

After reading this chapter, the student should be able to:

38.1 Describe the various respiratory diseases and conditions.

38.2 List signs and symptoms of respiratory complications of the various conditions.

38.3 Discuss proper stress reduction protocol measures for the respiratory patient.

38.4 Discuss proper management during a respiratory medical emergency.

38.5 Explain respiratory medications' mechanisms of action, potential side effects, and drug interactions.

38.6 Identify what patient interview questions regarding respiratory conditions are important for education, referral, and/or treatment alterations.

KEY CONCEPTS

• Respiratory pathogens responsible for acute respiratory infection reside in the oral cavity.

• Evaluation of health history, respiratory disease status, and medication usage, along with monitoring of vitals, are part of overall risk assessment for dental hygiene care.

• Precautions and treatment alterations for patients with respiratory disease need thorough consideration for prevention of respiratory complications and/or medical emergencies.

RELEVANCE TO CLINICAL PRACTICE

Respiratory diseases range from acute respiratory infections such as a cold, flu, or pneumonia to conditions such asthma and cystic fibrosis. Dental hygiene procedures can release oral bacteria that can be swallowed or inhaled and cause infection. They can also be stressful, which can exacerbate respiratory problems. To prevent respiratory complications and manage care appropriately, the dental hygienist should be able to: (1) recognize the signs and symptoms of the various respiratory diseases and conditions; (2) understand the actions, side effects, and drug interactions of respiratory medications; and (3) implement stress reduction protocol measures.

The Basics

1. All of the following are part of the lower tract of the respiratory system *except* for one. Which one is the *exception?*
   A. Bronchial tree
   B. Lungs
   C. Pharynx
   D. Trachea

2. Which type of asthma is triggered by allergens?
   A. Drug-induced
   B. Extrinsic
   C. Infectious
   D. Intrinsic

3. List the oral symptoms related to asthma inhaler use.

   1) _____

   2) _____

   3) _____

   4) _____

4. Choose all of the characteristics that apply to patients with emphysema.
   1) Tend to be cyanotic.
   2) Sometimes referred to as a "blue bloater."
   3) Tend to be barrel chested.
   4) Sometimes referred to as a "pink puffer."
      A. 1 and 2
      B. 1 and 4
      C. 2 and 3
      D. 3 and 4

5. Identify the medication that is associated with impaired healing.
   A. Fluticasone proprionate
   B. Montelukast
   C. Prednisone
   D. Theophylline

6. How can the extent and severity of respiratory disease be determined?

   _____

   _____

7. Select the classification for albuterol.
   A. Antileukotriene
   B. Corticosteroid
   C. Long-acting bronchodilator
   D. Short-acting bronchodilator

8. Identify the measurement of lung functioning capacity that signifies mild disease.
   A. Less than 60% forced expiratory volume (FEV)
   B. Greater than 80% FEV
   C. Less than 91% PO_2
   D. Greater than 95% PO_2

9. Which condition is classified as a lower respiratory tract infection?
   A. Common cold
   B. Influenza
   C. Pneumonia
   D. Strep throat

10. Identify the symptoms of acute respiratory disease.
    A. Cough lasting greater than 3 weeks
    B. Cough lasting less than 3 weeks
    C. Recurrent cough
    D. Noncommunicable

Learning Activities

1. Consider a patient who has been diagnosed with asthma. Discuss common allergens that may trigger a drug-induced asthma attack.

   _____

   _____

   _____

   _____

2. Your patient has recently been diagnosed with asthma and is using an albuterol inhaler. What advice should you provide to your patient?

   _____

   _____

   _____

   _____

Board Style Review Questions

1. Screening for tuberculosis includes a skin test called purified protein derivative (PPD). A positive PPD skin test shows immunity and requires no additional treatment.
   A. Both statements are true.
   B. The first statement is true; the second statement is false.
   C. Both statements are false.
   D. The first statement is false; the second statement is true.

2. What does pulse oximetry measure?
   A. Arterial blood oxygen saturation levels.
   B. Forced expiratory volume.
   C. Sputum and dyspnea.
   D. Forced expiratory volume in 1 second.

3. Identify the chronic lung disease characterized by inflammation and narrowing of the tracheobronchial tree.
   A. Asthma
   B. Chronic obstructive pulmonary disease
   C. Cystic fibrosis
   D. Tuberculosis

4. Choose the drug that is contraindicated for a patient taking erythromycin.
   A. Albuterol
   B. Corticosteroid
   C. Formoterol
   D. Theophylline

5. The upper tract of the respiratory system includes the:
   1) Lungs
   2) Oral cavity
   3) Pharynx
   4) Trachea
      A. 1 and 3
      B. 2 and 3
      C. 3 and 4
      D. 1, 2, and 3

6. Which type of asthma is associated with elevated serum immunoglobulin (IgE)?
   A. Drug-induced
   B. Extrinsic
   C. Infectious
   D. Intrinsic

7. Select the best definition for cystic fibrosis.
   A. Production of thick, sticky, mucus that causes blockage in the airway making it difficult to breath.
   B. Irreversible disease that obstructs airflow from the lungs and is both preventable and treatable.
   C. Chronic lung disease characterized by inflammation and narrowing of the tracheobronchial tree.
   D. Infectious and communicable pulmonary disease.

8. Identify the incorrect statement regarding tuberculosis (TB).
   A. It is a bloodborne pathogen.
   B. Infection can be present without symptoms.
   C. Individuals with tuberculosis have significant symptoms causing extreme disease.
   D. Individuals at higher risk include those who travel internationally, anyone in close contact with an infected individual, and/or immunocompromised individuals.

9. Select the appropriate course of action if your patient has a partial pressure of oxygen (PO_2) of 92%.
   A. No treatment change is necessary.
   B. Proceed with treatment and continue to monitor oxygen levels.
   C. Administer supplemental oxygen.
   D. Postpone treatment.

10. All of the following are considered inhaled short acting bronchodilators *except* for one. Which one is the *exception?*
    A. Albuterol
    B. Bitolterol mesylate
    C. Formoterol
    D. Pirbuterol

Chapter 39 | Sensory Disability: Vision and Hearing Impairment

KEY TERMS

American Sign
  Language (ASL)

blind

cataract

cochlear implant

deaf

diabetic retinopathy

finger spelling (American
  Manual Alphabet)

glaucoma

guide dog

hearing aid

hearing dog

legal blindness

lipreading

macular degeneration

service animal

tactile finger spelling

tactile sign
  language (TSL)

telecommunications
  device for the deaf
  (TDD)

teletypewriter (TTY)

tinnitus

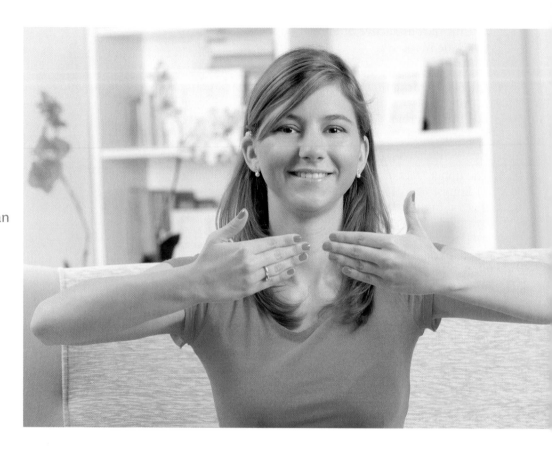

LEARNING OBJECTIVES

After reading this chapter, the student should be able to:

39.1 Describe blindness, low vision, and deafness.

39.2 Analyze the incidence of visual impairment in the United States.

39.3 Recognize the causes of blindness and hearing loss.

39.4 Identify the signs and types of hearing loss before and after birth and factors that contribute to lack of speech.

39.5 Distinguish the oral clinical findings commonly found in persons with sensory impairments.

39.6 Examine the personal and dental implications for care of patients with sensory impairments.

39.7 Explore strategies to communicate effectively with patients who have visual and hearing impairments.

39.8 Role-play seating and dismissal for the patient with visual impairment.

39.9 Develop management protocol that will enable you to provide safe and effective care for the patient with sensory impairments.

39.10 Plan an oral self-care program to improve the oral health of your patient with a sensory impairment.

KEY CONCEPTS

- Sensory disabilities alone do not require a change in treatment methods, just modifications in its provision.
- Sensory impairments alone have no direct effects on oral health; however, in patients with disabilities, there may be a greater incidence of dental disease because of lack of knowledge and communication about oral self-care or because of limited access.
- The Americans with Disabilities Act requires medical and dental offices to be made free of barriers to physical access and effective communication.
- Always ask patients with sensory disabilities what method of communication they prefer.
- Persons with sensory disabilities tend to rely more on their other senses.
- To prevent injury, ensure that the path to the dental operatory and the operatory itself are free of obstacles.
- Persons with a hearing disability may also have problems with speech.
- Appointments for patients with sensory impairments require extra time.
- Touch via hands is the primary method of communication for the person who is deaf and blind.

RELEVANCE TO CLINICAL PRACTICE

More than 20 million Americans report having loss of vision, including those who have trouble seeing even when wearing glasses or contact lenses, and those who are **blind,** or unable to see at all. Of those 20 million Americans, 6.2 million are seniors aged 65 years and older.[1] According to current U.S. Census Bureau Newsroom statistics, 1.8 million people aged 15 years and older report being unable to see printed words.[2] These figures translate to 1 of 20 dental patients having some degree of visual impairment.

Hearing impairment is often referred to as the invisible disability because there may be no visual clues that the person has an impairment. According to research studies, 35 million Americans are hearing impaired, corresponding to 11.3% of the U.S. population. Although hearing loss is considered a disability of the older adult, studies show that about 1 American school-aged child in 10 suffers from some form of hearing loss.[3] Those with hearing impairment are as individual as the cause and manifestation of their disability. Loss of function can be total or partial, affect one or both ears, and often impacts speech, language development, and even motor activity; communication is often a major challenge.[4] Many older persons have some degree of hearing impairment. As the baby boom generation (those born between 1946 and 1964) ages, the number of persons with vision and hearing loss will increase substantially.[5]

It is important for dental professionals to recognize the mental and physical aspects of having a sensory disability to use their resources and imagination to help furnish care. Sensory disabilities alone do not require a change in treatment methods, just modifications in its provision. Title III of the 1992 Americans with Disabilities Act requires medical and dental offices to be made free of barriers to physical access and effective communication.[6] Removing barriers for a blind person may involve adding raised letters or Braille to elevator control buttons, as well as providing written materials in Braille. For those with limited vision, the use of large-print materials is helpful. Effective communication for hearing-impaired persons may include auxiliary aids such as sign language interpreters, telecommunications devices such as a **teletypewriter (TTY)** for deaf persons, and the use of a reader.[6] Barriers to dental care for the patient with sensory impairments include physical access to the office, lack of transportation, lack of communication, and economic issues. Preparation, patience, flexibility, and consideration are essential and as valuable as technique in providing care.

The Basics

1. Which condition results from the rise of normal fluid pressure in the eye causing optic nerve damage?
   A. Diabetic retinopathy
   B. Cataracts
   C. Macular degeneration
   D. Glaucoma

2. All of the following are considerations for a patient with a hearing impairment *except* for one. Which one is the *exception*?
   A. The Americans with Disabilities Act mandates the use of an interpreter if the patient requires one.
   B. It is best to use a family member or friend to help with interpretation.
   C. The dental hygienist should ask the patient how he/she prefers to communicate.
   D. If an interpreter is used, the dental hygienist should talk directly to the patient who is deaf, not the interpreter.

3. List the communication options for a patient with hearing loss.

   1) _____

   2) _____

   3) _____

   4) _____

   5) _____

4. Usher's syndrome is:
   A. A genetic disorder causing deafness and blindness.
   B. An acquired disorder causing deafness and blindness.
   C. A genetic disorder causing hearing impairment.
   D. An acquired disorder causing visual impairment.

5. Report on the incidence of visual impairment in the United States.

_____

_____

_____

_____

_____

_____

_____

_____

6. Legal blindness is defined as visual acuity of:
   A. 20/200
   B. 20/20
   C. 20/10
   D. 20/100

7. When interacting with a guide dog or service animal, the dental hygienist should:
   A. Walk on the side opposite of the dog
   B. Offer the dog a treat
   C. Leave the dog outside the building until the patient is ready to leave
   D. Pet the guide dog so he/she becomes familiar with you

8. Title III of the 1992 Americans with Disabilities Act requires dental offices to be made free of barriers to physical access and effective communication. What barriers should be addressed for a person who is blind?

_____

_____

_____

_____

_____

_____

9. Identify four barriers to dental care for the patient with sensory impairments.

   1) _____   3) _____

   2) _____   4) _____

Learning Activities

1. Discuss with a student partner potential signs that a patient with a hearing impairment may exhibit.

_____

_____

_____

_____

_____

_____

2. Review the Americans with Disabilities Act. Consider a dental facility that you have recently visited. What modifications did the facility make to reduce barriers for patients with sensory impairments?

_____

_____

_____

_____

_____

_____

_____

_____

Board Style Review Questions

1. Which type of hearing loss involves the inner ear?
   1) Cochlear
   2) Conductive
   3) Sensorineural
      A. 1 and 2
      B. 1 and 3
      C. 2 and 3
      D. Only 2

2. A normal conversation occurs at:
   A. 100 decibels
   B. 85 decibels
   C. 60 decibels
   D. 40 decibels

3. Which condition affects the center of the visual field?
   A. Cataracts
   B. Diabetic retinopathy
   C. Glaucoma
   D. Macular degeneration

4. Which type of hearing loss reduces or distorts sound?
   A. Cochlear
   B. Conductive
   C. Sensorineural

5. A constant glare in the path of vision, double vision, and sensitivity to light are symptoms of which condition?
   A. Glaucoma
   B. Macular degeneration
   C. Cataract
   D. Strabismus

6. Incidence of dental disease may be greater due to:
   A. Poor oral self-care
   B. Vision impairment
   C. Hearing impairment
   D. Both vision and hearing loss

7. A cochlear implant can be used for patients who cannot be helped by hearing aids. This implant is an electronic device that restores normal hearing through a microphone and speech processor.
   A. Both statements are correct.
   B. The first statement is correct; the second is incorrect.
   C. Both statements are incorrect.
   D. To use a slow speed, heavier pressure, and wet prophy paste.

8. Which of following is not recommended when interacting with a patient who is using lipreading for communication?
   A. Stand in front of a light source
   B. Place the patient in the upright position
   C. Remove your mask
   D. Avoid turning your back when speaking

9. An impairment that results in a cloud that develops over the lens of the eye:
   A. Amblyopia
   B. Cataracts
   C. Glaucoma
   D. Strabismus

10. The term tinnitus can be described as:
    A. Visual impairment from damage to the optic nerve
    B. A degree of hearing loss
    C. Perception of sound or ringing in the ears
    D. An auxiliary aid

REFERENCES

1. Facts and figures about blind & visually impaired individuals in the US. American Foundation for the Blind website. http://www.afb.org/Section.asp?SectionID=15&DocumentID=4398#numbers. Accessed December 2010.
2. Facts for features: 20th anniversary of Americans with Disabilities Act: July 26. U.S. Census Bureau website.
3. 35 million Americans suffering from hearing loss. Hear-it.org website. http://www.hear-it.org/page.dsp?area=858. Accessed December 2010.
4. Dougal A, Fiske J. Access to special care dentistry, part 2. Communication. *Br Dent J.* 2008;205:11-21
5. Macera L. Preparing for the baby boomer generation. Geriatr Nurs. November/December 2007:46-49. National Student Nurses website. http://www.nsa.org. http://www.nsna.org/Portals/0/Skins/NSNA/pdf/Imprint_NovDec07_Feat_Geriatric.pdf. Accessed Oct. 9, 2015.
6. Americans with Disabilities Act. U.S. Department of Justice website. http://www.ada.gov/t3hilght.htm. Accessed May 2009.

Rubrics/Process Evaluations

Process Evaluation Template		
Dental Management of the Patient with Visual Impairment		
Evaluation Criteria	**Criteria Met? (Y/N)**	**Comments**
Student checks passages to ensure they are clear from clutter. (No loose rugs, hanging plants, etc.)		
Student identifies self and asks if the patient needs help.		
Student provides proper guidance to patient. (Instructs patient to take bent arm near elbow, avoids sudden/ unexpected movements, etc.)		
Patient seating. Student places the patient's hand on the back of the chair, stands near chair to assist as needed, gives a verbal description of where the chair is located.		
Student warns patient before adjusting the dental chair.		
If the glasses are removed, the student returns them to the patient before using any visual aids. If a light sensitivity exists, the student provides dark glasses.		
The student explains every procedure slowly using descriptive words, as well as describing smell and taste.		
Student avoids surprise applications of suction, air, water, etc.		
Discusses rinsing options.		
Student reverses seating procedures for patient dismissal and guides patient as necessary.		

Rubrics/Process Evaluations

Process Evaluation Template

Dental Management of the Patient with Hearing Impairment

Evaluation Criteria	Criteria Met? (Y/N)	Comments
Student summons the patient to the operatory by going out to the reception area rather than calling out the patient's name.		
Student keeps background noise to a minimum (radio, traffic noise, etc.).		
Student removes facemask to facilitate lipreading as needed.		
Student asks the patient if it is acceptable to use a gentle tap on the hand or arm to get his/her attention.		
Student explains each procedure and repeats or rephrases sentences so that the patient understands.		
Student demonstrates instruments and equipment as necessary.		
Student advises the patient to turn on a hearing aid for conversations and to turn it off when power-driven instruments are used.		
Uses standard precautions during procedure.		

Chapter 40 | Mental Health

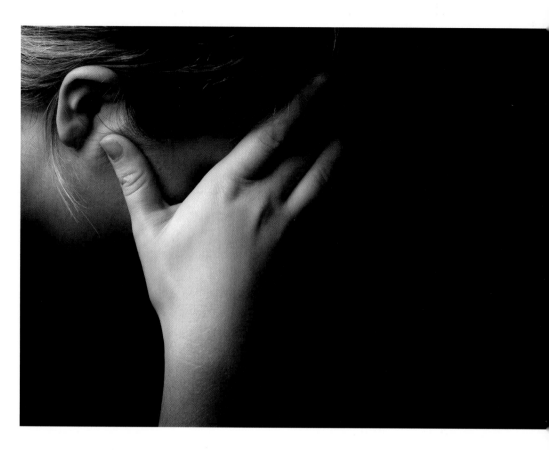

LEARNING OBJECTIVES

After reading this chapter, the student should be able to:

40.1 Describe the common mental disorders that may be encountered in dental hygiene care.

40.2 Discuss the implications of mental disorders on oral health.

40.3 Identify the common oral and dental manifestations of the mental disorders discussed.

40.4 Identify common oral manifestations associated with alcohol and illicit substance abuse.

40.5 Recognize the regularly prescribed medications for the mental disorders discussed and the oral/dental side effects.

40.6 Identify treatment preparation and planning modifications for patients with various mental disorders.

KEY CONCEPTS

• Evaluation of mental disabilities and psychiatric disorders as listed in patient medical histories is a part of risk assessment and treatment planning.

• There are treatment and home care modifications that should be made for patients with various mental disorders.

• It is essential for dental hygienists to identify common oral and dental issues that patients with mental disorders commonly have.

RELEVANCE TO CLINICAL PRACTICE

Twenty-one percent of Americans suffer from some form of mental disorder in any given year.[1,2] Mental disorders affect all age groups from early childhood to geriatric populations. Usually a direct correlation exists between these disabilities and poor oral health. The majority of patients suffering from mental disorders are also likely to be prescribed medications with oral side effects and dental treatment implications. As a dental hygienist, it is imperative to have a basic understanding of the behaviors and needs of patients with mental disorders that are likely to be encountered. Appropriate treatment modification and planning, with a strong focus on preventive measures, is key to the oral health of patients with mental disorders.

The Basics

1. Which of these conditions can best be described as a severe impairment in social interaction and communication?
   A. Autism spectrum disorder
   B. Dysthymic disorder
   C. Major depressive disorder (MDD)
   D. Schizophrenia

2. Leukoedema is an oral manifestation found more often among:
   A. Patients who abuse alcohol
   B. Patients who abuse cannabis
   C. Patients who abuse cocaine
   D. Patients who abuse methamphetamine
   E. Patients with schizophrenia

3. List potential oral manifestations associated with an eating disorder.

   1) _____

   2) _____

   3) _____

   4) _____

   5) _____

4. Xerostomia is an oral side effect of fluoxetine, paroxetine, and citalopram. All of these drugs are classified as:
   A. Anticonvulsants
   B. Antidepressants
   C. Antiepileptics
   D. CNS stimulants

5. Manic-depression is classified as:
   A. Dysthymic disorder
   B. Cyclothymic disorder
   C. Bipolar I disorder
   D. Bipolar II disorder

6. All of the following are mood disorders *except* for one. Which one is the *exception?*
   A. Bipolar disorders
   B. Dysthymic disorders
   C. Major depressive disorders
   D. Rhett's disorder

7. Long-term alcohol use causes swelling of the parotid gland. This swelling results in excess salivary flow.
   A. Both statements are true.
   B. The first statement is true; the second statement is false.
   C. Both statements are false.
   D. The first statement is false; the second statement is true.

8. Select the condition where people suffer from an acute occurrence of depression and exhibit symptoms severe enough to limit everyday normal functions.
   A. Autism
   B. Bipolar disorder
   C. Dysthymic disorder
   D. Major depressive disorder

9. Mood disorders are considered:
   A. Pervasive developmental disorders
   B. Disturbances in a person's emotional state
   C. Dangerous abnormalities in eating habits
   D. A more complicated risk to treatment due to resulting systemic effects

10. Extreme mood swings that fluctuate between euphoria and depression describes:
    A. Autism
    B. Bipolar disorder
    C. Dysthymic disorder
    D. Major depressive disorder

Learning Activities

1. Discuss the implications of mental disorders on oral health with a student partner.

_____

_____

_____

_____

_____

_____

_____

_____

_____

_____

_____

_____

2. Choose a commonly prescribed drug for treating mental disorders. Present key points and dental considerations to your classmates.

_____

_____

_____

_____

_____

_____

_____

_____

_____

_____

_____

_____

3. Identify dental hygiene considerations related to patients with autism spectrum disorders.

_____

_____

_____

_____

_____

_____

_____

_____

_____

_____

_____

_____

4. Design a visual aid, such as a flip chart, flash cards, or a storyboard, to outline the steps of a dental hygiene appointment. Use this to prepare your patients with autism for what to expect at his/her appointment.

Board Style Review Questions

1. Which of these best describes a condition associated with a very limited diet that favors soft, sugary foods?
   A. Schizophrenia
   B. Bulimia nervosa
   C. Autism spectrum disorder
   D. Anorexia nervosa

2. Which statement best characterizes Asperger's Syndrome?
   A. Disturbances in a person's mood or emotional state beyond what are considered normal.
   B. A condition classified as an autism spectrum disorder.
   C. Extreme mood swings between euphoria and depression.
   D. Odd physical behaviors or speech.

3. A patient who sees his/her body weight realistically, but fears gaining weight may suffer from:
   A. Anorexia nervosa
   B. Bulimia nervosa
   C. Schizophrenia
   D. Substance abuse

4. Suggested treatment considerations for a patient with autism spectrum disorder include all of the following *except* for one. Which one is the *exception?*
   A. Collaboration with the main caregiver.
   B. Preappointment visits to the office.
   C. Oral hygiene instructions for the caregiver.
   D. A rigid or structured appointment plan in order not to stress the patient with changes.

5. A patient who abuses cocaine may have which of the following oral/dental manifestations?
   1) Angular cheilosis
   2) Candidiasis
   3) Erosion
   4) Gold restoration erosion
      A. 1 and 2
      B. 2 and 3
      C. 1, 2, and 3
      D. 1, 2, and 4

6. All of the following are oral/dental manifestations of alcohol abuse *except* for one. Which one is the *exception?*
   A. Angular cheilosis
   B. Glossitis
   C. Bruxism
   D. Swollen parotid glands

7. Patients who abuse cannabis may exhibit which of the following oral/dental manifestations?
   1) Bruxism
   2) Leukoedema
   3) Leukoplakia
   4) Xerostomia
      A. 1, 2, and 3
      B. 2 and 3
      C. 2, 3, and 4
      D. Only 4

8. Tachycardia, confusion, and dilated pupils are manifestations of:
   A. Alcohol abuse
   B. Cocaine abuse
   C. Cannabis abuse
   D. Methamphetamine abuse

9. Which CNS stimulant is commonly prescribed for patients with autism?
   A. Ritalin
   B. Haldol
   C. Anafranil
   D. Adderall XR

10. You should avoid using epinephrine if your patient is on this drug:
    A. Celexa
    B. Clozaril
    C. Effexor
    D. Paxil

REFERENCES

1. Halgin, RP, Witbourne, SK *Abnormal Psychology: Clinical Perspectives on Psychological Disorders with DSM-5 update.* 7th Ed. New York: McGraw-Hill; 2013.
2. U.S. Department of Health and Human Services. *Mental Health: A Report of the Surgeon General—Executive Summary.* Rockville, MD: U.S. Department of Health and Human Services, Substance Abuse and Mental Health Services Administration, Center for Mental Health Services, National Institutes of Health, National Institute of Mental Health; 1999.

Chapter 41 | Neurological Impairments

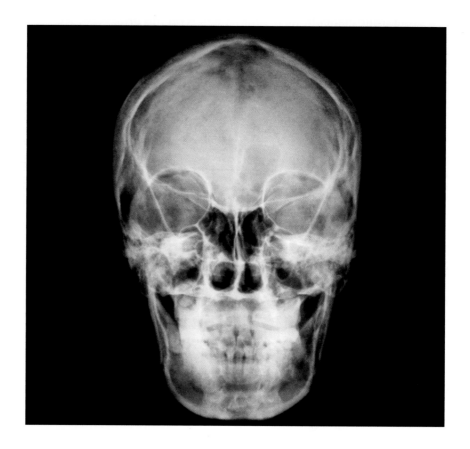

LEARNING OBJECTIVES

After reading this chapter, the student should be able to:

41.1 Identify the categories of neurological impairments.

41.2 Describe the common neurological impairments and their symptoms.

41.3 Identify common medications prescribed for neurological impairments including predominant contraindications or precautions, adverse reactions, and side effects.

41.4 Identify the effects of neurological impairments on the oral condition.

41.5 Assess patient/client needs based on data collection.

41.6 Develop an individualized treatment (care) plan including implementation strategies for modifications based on assessment of patient/client needs.

41.7 Develop individualized health-promoting goals and strategies for home care and maintenance.

41.8 Present and explain the home-care plan to the patient and caregiver.

KEY CONCEPTS

• Using critical thinking and sensitivity during the dental hygiene assessment is vital to developing adaptive methods of treatment delivery.

• Confidence in the dental hygienist's education and skill development enhances the comfort level of interacting and communicating with and treating the patient with neurological impairment.

- Modified treatment modalities maximize patient safety, comfort, and response.
- Interdisciplinary assessment and treatment planning results in comprehensive, total health outcomes.

RELEVANCE TO CLINICAL PRACTICE

Neurological disorders affect up to 1 billion people worldwide.[1] It is estimated that just more than 50 million Americans are affected by a neurological disorder, which equates to 1 in 6 people (World Health Organization [WHO], as reported by the American Academy of Neurology, A. Babb, Associate Director, Media and Public Relations, and D. Hoch, Department of Neurology, Massachusetts General Hospital, e-mail communication, September 2, 2010).[1] Some of the most common causes of neurological impairments are projected to increase substantially worldwide by the years 2017 and 2030.[1] Consequently, the number of patients with neurological impairments whom the dental hygienist will treat will also increase proportionately. The most recent survey results (2008) revealed that only 42% of dental hygiene programs require students to gain clinical experiences with patients with special needs.[2] It has and will become increasingly necessary for dental hygiene students to gain the experience and confidence in recognizing and treating patients with neurological impairments throughout the entire educational process. This chapter provides a comprehensive overview of the patient with neurological impairment and assists dental hygienists in developing a perspective of flexibility in modifying and adapting treatment modalities based on their patient assessments (see Chapter 8) and needs. It also focuses on enhancing effective communication skills among the patient, provider, and caregiver.

The Basics

1. Neurological impairments are disorders of the peripheral nervous system. These impairments can be specific to the brain and specific to the spinal cord.
   A. Both statements are true.
   B. The first statement is true; the second statement is false.
   C. Both statements are false.
   D. The first statement is false; the second statement is true.

2. All of the following statements are true of amyotrophic lateral sclerosis (ALS) *except* for one. Which one is the *exception?*
   A. A neuromuscular disease that eventually results in death
   B. Referred to as Lou Gehrig's disease
   C. No specific therapy exists
   D. Median survival time from onset is 5 years

3. Spastic palsy is characterized by writhing movements. Dyskinetic palsy is characterized by stiff or rigid muscles.
   A. Both statements are correct.
   B. The first statement is correct; the second statement is incorrect.
   C. Both statements are incorrect.
   D. The first statement is incorrect; the second statement is correct.

4. After paralysis from Bell palsy, the facial muscles tend to become:
   A. Hypotonic
   B. Hypertonic
   C. Hypertrophic
   D. Hyperacusis

5. Select the most applicable dental hygiene consideration for a patient with myasthenia gravis.
   A. Provide sunglasses.
   B. Provide a writing pad.
   C. Use an attachable headrest with restraints.
   D. Ensure safety and comfort due to the rapid progression of the disease.

6. List the oral symptoms of Bell palsy.
   1) _____
   2) _____
   3) _____

7. Your patient has been diagnosed with multiple sclerosis. List three potential barriers to receiving dental hygiene care.
   1) _____
   2) _____
   3) _____

8. Patients with spastic palsy may develop an abnormal curvature of the spine referred to as:
   A. Asthenia
   B. Dysarthria
   C. Hyperacusis
   D. Scoliosis

9. Select the most applicable dental hygiene consideration for a patient with cerebral palsy.
   A. Provide sunglasses.
   B. Provide a writing pad.
   C. Use an attachable headrest with restraints.
   D. Ensure safety and comfort due to the rapid progression of the disease.

Learning Activities

1. Choose a neurological impairment and develop a case study to share with your class.

_____

_____

_____

_____

_____

_____

_____

_____

_____

_____

_____

_____

_____

_____

_____

_____

_____

_____

2. Select a neurological impairment and role-play with a student partner. Discuss the home-care plan with the patient and caregiver.

3. Explain how interdisciplinary assessment is important to health outcomes for patients with neurological impairments.

_____

_____

_____

_____

_____

_____

_____

_____

_____

_____

_____

_____

_____

_____

_____

_____

Board Style Review Questions

1. Match the following terms with the appropriate definition.

   _____ Akinesia   A. Speech or language deficits

   _____ Aphasia   B. Loss of half of visual field

   _____ Dysphonia   C. Short, shuffling steps

   _____ Festination   D. Muscle rigidity

   _____ Hemianopsia   E. Speaking or voice impairments

2. Chorea, dystonia, and dysphagia are symptoms of which condition:
   A. ALS
   B. Bell palsy
   C. Cerebral palsy
   D. Huntington disease

3. Neurological impairments specific to the brain include:
   1) Sleep and arousal disorders
   2) Respiration
   3) Motor disturbances
   4) Sensory disturbances
      A. 1 and 2
      B. 1, 2, and 3
      C. 1, 3, and 4
      D. 2, 3, and 4

4. All of the following impairments are specific to the spinal cord *except* for one. Which one is the *exception?*
   A. Station and gait
   B. Urinary bladder function
   C. Sexual function
   D. Emotional disturbances

5. Which of the following conditions is associated with herpes simplex or varicella virus infection?
   A. ALS
   B. Bell palsy
   C. Cerebral palsy
   D. Huntington disease

6. Chorea is defined as:
   A. Quick, dance-like, uncontrollable movements of the limbs.
   B. A constant writhing, twisting, uncontrollable movement.
   C. Difficulty in swallowing.
   D. Trembling during voluntary movement.

7. All of the following are dental hygiene considerations for treating a patient with Huntington disease *except* for one. Which one is the *exception?*
   A. Frequent application of fluoride varnish.
   B. Position patient in the upright position.
   C. Due to ambulatory limitations, a longer visit should be planned to complete all treatment.
   D. A mouth prop.

8. Impairments to bulbar muscles which manifest in facial or oropharyngeal muscle weakness are signs of:
   A. Bell palsy
   B. Cerebral palsy
   C. Myasthenia gravis
   D. Parkinson disease

9. A patient may be prescribed anticoagulants after a stroke. Which of the following can counteract the effects of warfarin?
   1) Vitamin C
   2) Vitamin K
   3) Tetracycline
      A. 1 and 2
      B. 1 and 3
      C. 2 and 3
      D. Only 3

10. Which of the following is characteristic of a stroke victim who experiences right hemispheric effects?
    A. Paralysis on the right side of the body
    B. Impulsive behavior
    C. Speech deficits
    D. Slow, cautious behavior

REFERENCES

1. World Health Organization (WHO)/Brussels/Geneva, News Release. Neurological disorders affect millions globally: WHO Report. Geneva, Switzerland: WHO; February 27, 2007.
2. Dehaitem M, Ridley K, Kerschbaum W, Inglehart M. Dental hygiene education about patients with special needs: a survey of U.S. programs. *J Dent Educ.* 2008;72(9):1010-1019.

Chapter 42 | Endocrine System

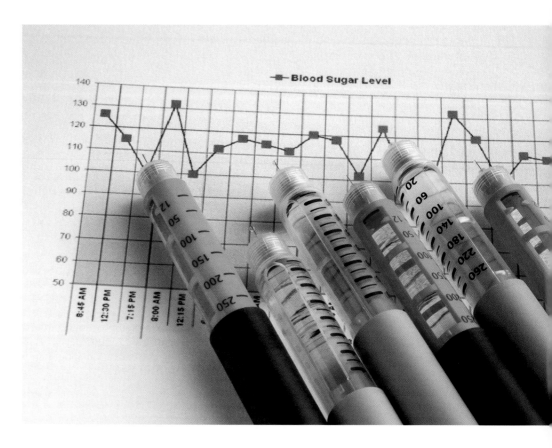

LEARNING OBJECTIVES

After reading this chapter, the student should be able to:

42.1 Identify endocrine system disorders most commonly encountered in dental hygiene practice.

42.2 Discuss the implications of endocrine disorders on oral health.

42.3 Develop individualized dental hygiene care plans for patients with endocrine disorders.

42.4 Implement the necessary dental hygiene treatment modifications for patients with various endocrine conditions.

KEY CONCEPTS

- The endocrine system is an important body health system with many complications.
- The diseases of the endocrine system have dental considerations.
- The dental hygienist must be aware of patients' medical health in relation to their oral health needs including periodontal disease and the oral–systemic connection.

RELEVANCE TO PRACTICE

The Centers for Disease Control and Prevention estimates that 29.1 million Americans, or 9.3% of the population, have diabetes. Of those people, 21.0 million have been diagnosed with diabetes and 8.1 million are undiagnosed. New cases of diabetes continue to be diagnosed, particularly among adults aged 45 years and older.[1] Patients with diabetes may also have other conditions, including periodontitis and hypertension. Links have been shown between diabetes and periodontitis. Diabetes is a risk factor for periodontitis, and periodontal inflammation negatively affects control of diabetes.[2] The National Diabetes Education Program recommends that dental professionals collaborate with primary care providers, nurses, diabetes educators, pharmacists, and other health-care professionals to provide patient-centered care to patients with diabetes.[3] For effective collaboration and positive patient outcomes, dental hygienists need to understand the diabetes disease process, its effect on the patient's oral health, and dental hygiene care modifications for the patient with diabetes.

Thyroid disorders are other common disorders of the endocrine system. It is estimated that 20 million Americans have a thyroid disorder, and more than 12% of Americans will experience development of a thyroid disorder.[4] Dental hygienists need to know how these diseases impact their patients' oral health and how to modify treatment for patients with these conditions.

The Basics

1. For patients with diabetes, an A_{1C} less than 7 is considered:
   A. Too low
   B. Acceptable
   C. Slightly elevated
   D. Moderately elevated

2. An iodine deficiency can lead to:
   A. Insufficient thyroid hormone production
   B. Excess growth hormone production
   C. A characteristic round or moon shaped face
   D. Increased blood glucose levels

3. Choose the best definition for Cushing disease.
   A. A disorder resulting from a lack of hormones from the adrenal medulla.
   B. A disorder caused from oversecretion of the parafollicular cells.
   C. A disorder that occurs when the body is exposed to high levels of cortisol.
   D. A disorder caused from excess growth hormone.

4. Your patient with diabetes had lunch 2 hours ago. Which of these glucose readings is within the target range for an after meal measurement?
   1) 130 mg/dL
   2) 142 mg/dL
   3) 179 mg/dL
   4) 188 mg/dL
      A. 1 and 2
      B. 1, 2, and 3
      C. All are within the target range.
      D. Only 1

5. Subgingival irrigation with 10% povidone-iodine can be used in combination with scaling and root planing. Which condition is not a contraindication for treatment with povidone-iodine?
   A. Thyroid pathosis
   B. Pregnancy
   C. Iodine hypersensitivity
   D. Acromegaly

6. List the symptoms of ketoacidosis.

   _____   _____

   _____   _____

7. The saliva of patients with diabetes can have high glucose levels. Provide two oral health concerns for high glucose levels in saliva.

   1) _____

   2) _____

8. Explain the role of glucagon when blood sugar levels start to fall.

   _____

   _____

   _____

   _____

   _____

   _____

   _____

9. The systolic blood pressure reading measures the pressure in the arteries when the heart is relaxed. A systolic reading greater than 140 mm Hg is classified as hypertension.
   A. Both statements are correct.
   B. The first statement is correct; the second statement is incorrect.
   C. Both statements are incorrect.
   D. The first statement is incorrect; the second statement is correct.

10. Describe where the thyroid is located.

    _____

    _____

    _____

    _____

    _____

    _____

Learning Activities

1. Role-play with a student partner. Call your patient's medical office to inquire about his/her health status.

2. Make a list of questions that the clinician should ask a patient with diabetes during review of the medical history.

_____

_____

_____

_____

_____

_____

_____

_____

_____

_____

_____

_____

_____

_____

_____

_____

_____

_____

_____

_____

_____

_____

Board Style Review Questions

1. All of the following statements are correct of type 1 diabetes _except_ for one. Which one is the _exception?_
   A. It is an autoimmune disorder.
   B. It may be triggered in a genetically susceptible individual.
   C. It must be treated with insulin.
   D. It is associated with obesity.

2. Choose the hormone action in which hormones cause a condition to intensify and not decrease.
   A. Direct nervous stimulation
   B. Negative feedback system
   C. Positive feedback system
   D. Tropic hormones

3. Which gland secretes melatonin?
   A. Adrenal
   B. Pineal
   C. Pituitary
   D. Thyroid

4. Define circadian rhythm.
   A. Regular changes in mental and physical characteristics that occur over the course of a day.
   B. Regulation of the activity of the glands in the body.
   C. Changes in hormone levels throughout the day.
   D. Regulation of nerve impulses and muscle contraction in the body.

5. Which hormone is secreted if blood calcium levels become too high?
   A. Adrenocorticotropic hormone (ACTH)
   B. Calcitonin
   C. Mineralocorticoids
   D. Triiodothyronine

6. The adrenal gland is divided into an outer adrenal cortex and an inner medulla. The medulla is essential to life but the adrenal cortex can be removed with no life-threatening effects.
   A. Both statements are true.
   B. The first statement is true; the second statement is false.
   C. Both statements are false.
   D. The first statement is false; the second statement is true.

7. What is (are) the function(s) of aldosterone?
   1) To maintain blood pressure and blood volume.
   2) To inhibit the amount of sodium excreted in the urine.
   3) To increase blood glucose levels.
   4) To help distribute body fat.
      A. 1 and 2
      B. 2 and 3
      C. 3 and 4
      D. Only 1

8. Identify the best descriptor of glycogen.
   A. A form of glucose secreted by the pancreas.
   B. A hormone secreted by the adrenal cortex.
   C. A hormone secreted by the beta cells in the pancreatic islets.
   D. A form of glucose that is stored in the liver.

9. Select the pre-meal healthy blood glucose range.
   A. Less than 70 mg/dL
   B. 70 to 130 mg/dL
   C. 130 to 180 mg/dL
   D. 140 to 180 mg/dL

10. Choose the term that signifies symptoms of increased appetite.
    A. Polymerization
    B. Polydipsia
    C. Polyuria
    D. Polyphagia

Active Learning

Your patient presents for dental hygiene care. She has a history of type 1 diabetes and reports having taken her insulin 30 minutes before the appointment with her breakfast. After reviewing her histories and completing her assessments, you notice that she is sweating and she says she does not feel well.

1. The dental hygienist should:
   A. Administer oxygen
   B. Provide the patient with water or a sugar-free beverage to address dehydration
   C. Provide an antihypoglycemic
   D. Have the patient administer a dose of insulin

2. This patient has the type of diabetes that:
   A. Is associated with obesity
   B. Is not autoimmune
   C. Produces insulin but the cells cannot respond normally
   D. Causes the immune system to destroy insulin-producing beta cells

3. Identify the most appropriate protocol that could have been implemented to avoid this type of medical emergency.
   A. The patient should not have been scheduled for treatment during peak insulin activity.
   B. The patient should have avoided carbohydrate intake before the appointment.
   C. Blood pressure should have been assessed.
   D. The patient should not have administered a dose of insulin before the appointment.

REFERENCES

1. National Diabetes Statistics Report, 2014. Atlanta, GA: Centers for Disease Control and Prevention. http://www.cdc.gov/diabetes/pubs/statsreport14/national-diabetes-report-web.pdf. Accessed October 3, 2015.
2. Preshaw PM, Alba AL, Herrara D, et al. Periodontitis and diabetes: a two-way relationship. *Diabetologia*. 2012;55(1):21-31. http://www.ncbi.nlm.nih.gov/pmc/articles/PMC3228943. Accessed October 3, 2015.
3. What makes a team? Bethesda, MD: National Institute of Diabetes and Digestive and Kidney Diseases. http://ndep.nih.gov/hcp-businesses-and-schools/practice-transformation/team-based-care/what-makes-a-team.aspx. Accessed October 3, 2015.
4. General information/press room. Falls Church, VA: American Thyroid Association. http://www.thyroid.org/media-main/about-hypothyroidism. Updated 2014. Accessed October 3, 2015.

Chapter 43 | Immune System

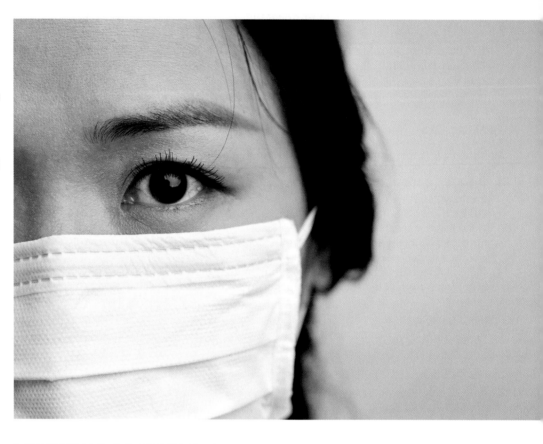

LEARNING OBJECTIVES

After reading this chapter, the student should be able to:

43.1 Discuss the general concepts of human immunity.

43.2 Describe the effects of each presented disease on general and oral health.

43.3 Identify precautions and modifications to dental hygiene care for each presented disease.

43.4 Critically evaluate a patient's medical history and list of medications in preparation for treating a patient with immune system dysfunction.

43.5 Provide safe and effective care for patients with immune system dysfunction.

multiple sclerosis (MS)

myasthenia gravis (MG)

myasthenic crisis

palliative

paroxysmal pain
   syndromes

plasmapheresis

pleurisy

Raynaud phenomenon

rheumatoid arthritis (RA)

scleroderma (SC)

Sjögren syndrome (SS)

spasticity

systemic lupus
   erythematosus (SLE)

thymectomy

Wickham striae

xerophthalmia

KEY CONCEPTS

- Immune system dysfunction affects the patient's overall health, as well as their oral health.
- It is necessary for the dental hygienist to understand the progression and characteristics of a disease to safely treat a patient with immune dysfunction.
- Evaluation of the medical history and medications is part of the assessment phase of dental hygiene treatment.
- Appropriate treatment modification for patients with immune dysfunction is a critical part of both the planning and the implementation phases of dental hygiene treatment.

RELEVANCE TO CLINICAL PRACTICE

Dental hygienists in clinical practice will see a wide variety of patients, typically ranging from the very young to the very old. Many of those patients will have some form of immune system disorder. Autoimmune diseases, immune complex diseases, and immunodeficiency diseases all negatively affect the performance of the immune system. Because these diseases are relatively common among the population at large, it is very important for the clinician to have a thorough understanding of how they affect the body, what types of treatments are available, and what modifications may be necessary for treatment planning and patient recommendations.

The Basics

1. Substances that the immune system identifies as nonself are know as:
   A. Antibodies
   B. Antigens
   C. Autoimmune
   D. Immunoglobulins

2. All of the following are defense mechanisms of the innate immune system *except* for one. Which one is the *exception?*
   A. Acidity of stomach fluid
   B. B cells of the islets of Langerhans
   C. Skin and mucous membranes
   D. Urine

3. Which of the following are white blood cells?
   1) Cytokines
   2) B lymphocytes
   3) T lymphocytes
      A. 1 and 2
      B. 1 and 3
      C. 2 and 3
      D. Only 1

4. Phagocytes that circulate in the blood before they enter the tissue are called:
   A. Granulocytes
   B. Macrophages
   C. Monocytes
   D. Natural killer cells

5. Widening of the periodontal ligament space of all teeth with no evidence of occlusal trauma may be indicative of:
   A. Type 1 diabetes
   B. scleroderma
   C. myasthenia gravis
   D. Sjögren syndrome

6. Proteins made by cells that affect the behavior of other cells are:
   A. Helper T cells
   B. Natural killer cells
   C. Cytokines
   D. Chemokines

7. All of the following relate to immunodeficiency *except* for one. Which one is the *exception?*
   A. Missing or dysfunctional components of the immune system
   B. Caused by genetic mutation or by pathogens
   C. Acquired immune deficiency syndrome (AIDS)
   D. Type 1 diabetes

8. Salivary gland swelling can be an external sign of salivary dysfunction and is most common among patients with:
   A. Sjögren syndrome
   B. Scleroderma
   C. Myasthenia gravis
   D. Multiple sclerosis

Learning Activities

1. Create a chart of the immune system disorders. Specify the pathogenesis, treatment, and effects on oral health/dental considerations for each disorder.

2. Outline the basic concepts of immunity using the provided tree graph.

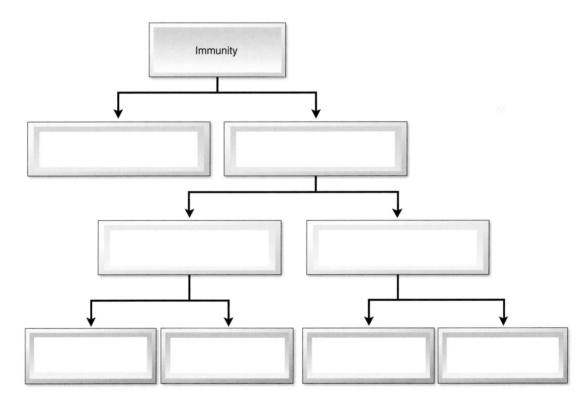

Board Style Review Questions

1. Powered scalers and air polishers are contraindicated for use on patients with which condition?
   A. Addison's disease
   B. Fibromyalgia
   C. Scleroderma
   D. Stevens-Johnson

2. An autoimmune disease that results in pain, swelling, and loss of function in the joints describes which condition?
   A. Addison's disease
   B. Fibromyalgia
   C. Multiple sclerosis
   D. Rheumatoid arthritis

3. Treatment of multiple sclerosis may include all of the following *except* for one. Which one is the *exception?*
   A. Prednisone
   B. Beta interferons
   C. Cholinesterase inhibitors
   D. Methylprednisolone

4. Red skin rashes called Malar or butterfly rash are associated with:
   A. Addison's disease
   B. Systemic lupus erythematosus
   C. Rheumatoid arthritis
   D. Scleroderma

5. Which of the following is a sign of Addisonian crisis?
   A. Sensations of prickling or pins and needles
   B. Spasticity
   C. Paroxysmal pain syndrome
   D. Dropping blood pressure

6. Cortisol functions to:
   1) Maintain blood glucose levels
   2) Maintain blood pressure
   3) Regulate salt/water balance
   4) Influence kidneys to excrete potassium
      A. 1 and 2
      B. 1 and 3
      C. 2 and 3
      D. 2 and 4

7. Fibromyalgia (FM) is a disorder that causes muscle pain and fatigue. The etiology of FM is unknown.
   A. Both statements are true.
   B. The first statement is true; the second statement is false.
   C. Both statements are false.
   D. The first statement is false; the second statement is true.

8. AIDS is diagnosed when the patient has a CD4+ count of?
   A. Less than 100 cells/mm^3
   B. Less than 200 cells/mm^3
   C. Less than 300 cells/mm^3
   D. Less than 400 cells/mm^3

9. A network of lines that are lacy in appearance called Wickham striae characterize lesions from lichen planus. These lesions are asymmetrical.
   A. Both statements are correct.
   B. The first statement is correct; the second statement is incorrect.
   C. Both statements are incorrect.
   D. The first statement is incorrect; the second statement is correct.

10. Medications approved by the Food and Drug Administration (FDA) for the treatment of fibromyalgia include all of the following *except* for one. Which one is the *exception?*
    A. Cymbalta
    B. Jentadueto
    C. Lyrica
    D. Savella

Chapter 44 | Hematological Considerations

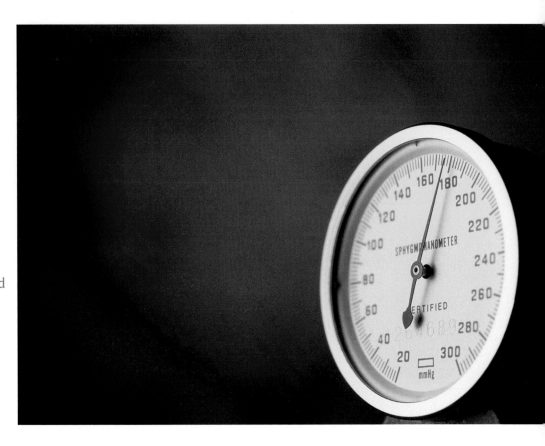

LEARNING OBJECTIVES

After reading this chapter, the student should be able to:

44.1 Identify medical conditions associated with increased bleeding.

44.2 Define types of bleeding disorders.

44.3 Determine whether treatment modifications are necessary for conditions with increased bleeding.

44.4 Identify medications that affect clotting.

44.5 Describe the management of a hematological emergency in the dental hygiene services.

44.6 Differentiate between red blood cell disorders and white blood cell disorders.

KEY CONCEPTS

• All individuals have the right to seek treatment for their dental needs. It is the responsibility of the dental team to determine how best to manage any individual who presents with health considerations.

• The dental team collaborates with other health-care practitioners to offer the best possible treatment. Understanding how the body's clotting mechanism works, what various laboratory values might indicate, their potential complications, and how to manage complications will ensure proper care and reduce the risk of an emergency.

- When treating patients with hematological conditions, the dental hygienist considers what the patient needs to do before the appointment, what the hygienist needs to do (treatment considerations) before the appointment, whether the hygienist can identify warning signs that would affect management of the dental hygiene appointment, and what the protocols are for handling an emergency with a patient who has a hematological condition.

RELEVANCE TO CLINICAL PRACTICE

The body is a complex system of organs and other tissues maintained by the hematological system. The human body would not be able to sustain itself if it were not for the complex "highways" of veins and arteries that provide needed nutrients to all of the organs in the body. Although it is very complex, the purpose of the hematological system is very simple: to transport nutrients to the organs in the body (through the arteries) and transport waste out (via the veins). Should injury occur anywhere along its many pathways, the body's defense mechanism is the formation of blood clots that help to slow down and stop the flow of blood out of the injured blood vessel. Blood clotting is a critical factor in ensuring the survival of the individual. Blood clotting is influenced by conditions such as blood disorders, bone marrow disorders, and blood diseases, as well as medications. Dental hygienists need to understand clotting principles and how various conditions and medications may affect clotting to plan and implement appropriate dental hygiene services for patients.[1]

The Basics

1. What is an appropriate International Normalized Ratio (INR) for a patient taking anticoagulants?
    A. 1.0
    B. 2.0 to 3.0
    C. 3.0 to 4.0
    D. 4.0

2. Choose the best term. Bone marrow is responsible for the formation of:
    A. Clots
    B. Clumps
    C. Fibrin
    D. Platelets

3. The platelets form clumps, continuously attaching to each other. These formations of clumps are known as:
    A. Fibrin
    B. Platelets
    C. Prothrombin
    D. White clots

4. Changes in filiform papillae may result from a deficiency in which of these nutrients?
   1) Vitamin B$_{12}$
   2) Vitamin K
   3) Folic acid
   4) Iron
      A. 1 and 2
      B. 1 and 4
      C. 2 and 3
      D. 3 and 4

5. Which of these tests does not determine bleeding time?
   A. INR
   B. Partial thromboplastin time (PTT)
   C. Prothrombin time
   D. Complete blood count (CBC)

6. Select the normal range of hemoglobin for females.
   A. 33% to 43%
   B. 39% to 49%
   C. 12 to 15 g/100 mL
   D. 13.6 to 17.2 g/100 mL

7. Which of these blood-thinning drugs is a vitamin K antagonist?
   A. Acetylsalicylic acid
   B. Aspirin
   C. Plavix
   D. Warfarin

8. Identify the blood count that represents thrombocytopenia.
   A. Less than 150,000 cells/mm
   B. 50,000 to 60,000 cells/mm
   C. 150,000 to 400,000 cells/mm
   D. Greater than 400,000 cells/mm

9. The lower the INR, the longer it takes blood to clot. It takes the average person 1 to 6 minutes to clot.
   A. Both statements are correct.
   B. The first statement is correct; the second statement is incorrect.
   C. Both statements are incorrect.
   D. The first statement is incorrect; the second statement is correct.

10. Which level of the PTT signifies a severe bleeding problem?
    A. Less than 50 sec
    B. Greater than 50 sec
    C. 11 to 16 sec
    D. 25 to 40 sec

Learning Activities

1. Explain to a classmate why physicians prefer the INR test to the prothrombin time (PT) test.

_____

_____

_____

_____

_____

_____

_____

_____

_____

_____

2. In small groups, describe the process for handling a hematological emergency.

_____

_____

_____

_____

_____

_____

_____

_____

_____

_____

_____

3. Make a checklist of each hematological condition. Determine when a medical consultation with the patient's physician is necessary. For each condition, what are the dental hygiene considerations?

_____

_____

_____

_____

_____

_____

_____

_____

_____

_____

Board Style Review Questions

1. A complete blood count (CBC) test can determine whether blood clotting is normal. The CBC assesses red blood cells, white blood cells, and platelets.
   A. Both statements are true.
   B. The first statement is true; the second statement is false.
   C. Both statements are false.
   D. The first statement is false; the second statement is true.

2. Choose the best description for polycythemia.
   A. Reduced production of red blood cells.
   B. Uncontrolled growth of B lymphocytes.
   C. Overproduction of red blood cells.
   D. Inflammation of the liver caused by a virus.

3. Identify the most transmissible form of hepatitis.
   A. Hepatitis B
   B. Hepatitis C
   C. Hepatitis D
   D. Hepatitis non-ABCDE

4. Which inherited bleeding disorder results from a missing or reduced protein needed to form blood clots?
   A. Anemia
   B. Hemophilia A
   C. Hemophilia B
   D. von Willebrand disease

5. Identify the drug that both inhibits long-term thrombus formation and causes short-term vasodilation.
   A. Aggrenox
   B. Dipyridamole
   C. Plavix
   D. Pradaxa

6. Which type of hepatitis infection occurs during blood transfusions?
   A. Hepatitis B
   B. Hepatitis C
   C. Hepatitis D
   D. Hepatitis non-ABCDE

7. Identify the nutrient that when deficient can cause anemia associated with a bluish tint in the whites of the eyes.
   A. Folic acid
   B. Iron
   C. Vitamin B_{12}
   D. Vitamin K

8. Your patient presents with an INR count of 4.0. Identify the appropriate course of treatment.
   A. Limit dental hygiene treatment to prophylaxis; do not perform scaling and root planing (SRP) procedures.
   B. Proceed with treatment but monitor bleeding.
   C. Do not provide treatment.
   D. Proceed with treatment; no changes to treatment are necessary.

9. Select the blood count level that represents thrombocytopenia.
   A. 25 to 40 sec
   B. Greater than 50 sec
   C. 150,000 cells/mm or less
   D. 150,000 to 400,000 cells/mm

10. On review of the radiographs, the dental hygienist notices a loss of trabeculation and large, irregular-shaped spaces of marrow loss. These signs are suggestive of which condition?
    A. Celiac sprue
    B. Pernicious anemia
    C. Sickle cell anemia
    D. Vitamin B_{12} deficiency

REFERENCES

1. Ibsen OAC, Phelan JA. Oral manifestations of systemic disease. In: Ibsen OAC, Phelan JA, eds. *Oral Pathology for the Dental Hygienist.* 6th ed. St. Louis, MO: Saunders Elsevier; 2014:282-296.

Chapter 45 | Cancer

KEY TERMS

adjunctive screening
  techniques

cancer

chemotherapy

field cancerization

metastasis

mucositis

multidisciplinary
  team (MDT)

nadir

oral squamous cell
  carcinoma (OSCC)

osteoradionecrosis (ORN)

radiation caries

risk factor

salivary diagnostics

tumor

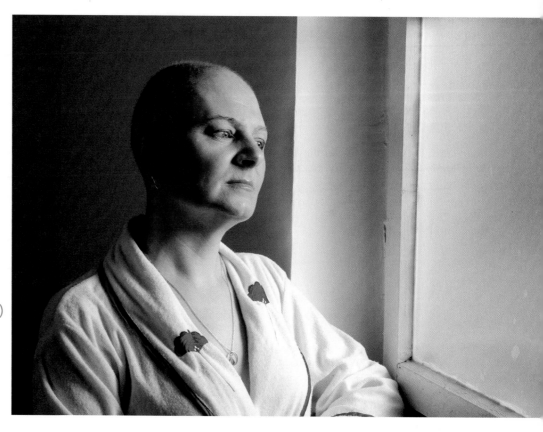

LEARNING OBJECTIVES

After reading this chapter, the student should be able to:

45.1 Define the terms *cancer* and *staging*, and explain how cancer is staged.

45.2 Discuss the incidence, risk factors, therapies, and potential oral complications related to treatment for all cancers.

45.3 Discuss the incidence, risk factors, therapies, and oral complications unique to head and neck cancers.

45.4 Identify behavioral interventions recommended for reducing the incidence of oral cancer.

45.5 Identify the common signs and symptoms of oral cancer.

45.6 Discuss dental hygiene care plan treatment alterations or precautions to be taken with patients with cancer.

KEY CONCEPTS

• Risk assessment for cancer is a critical part of comprehensive health care for all patients.

• Dental hygiene care of patients with cancer requires individualized consideration of systemic and oral complications.

• Types of treatment for cancer and oral cancer include chemotherapy, radiation therapy, surgery, and/or bone marrow and stem cell transplantation, all of which require consideration of precautions in dental hygiene care.

RELEVANCE TO CLINICAL PRACTICE

Because of improvements in health care and asepsis, expected life span is increasing worldwide. Along with this longer life expectancy, the incidence of cancer has increased over the past 50 years. **Cancer** is a general term that applies to a group of more than 100 diseases in which cells in a part of the body begin to grow out of control. Although there are many kinds of cancer, they all start because these abnormal cells proliferate uncontrollably. Untreated cancers can cause serious illness and even death.[1] Early detection and treatment should reduce mortality rate and morbidity from cancers and their treatment. Cancer care can be complex, and more recently, it is being directed by a **multidisciplinary team (MDT)** of health-care professionals. People cared for by a MDT are more likely to: (a) receive accurate diagnosis and staging, (b) be offered a choice of treatments, (c) receive appropriate and consistent information, and (d) have their psychological and social needs considered.[2] The dental hygienist can play an important role on that team. Treatment improvements are largely directed at targeted therapy designed to treat the cancer cells with minimal effects on healthy cells; however, reducing complications from treatment remains a major issue in both general cancers of the body and those specific to oral cancer.

The Basics

1. The most common opportunistic infection of the oropharynx in irradiated patients is:
   A. *Candida*
   B. Dysgeusia
   C. Herpes simplex
   D. Mucositis
   E. Peritonsillar abscess

2. The most common acute complication following chemotherapy is:
   A. Periodontal disease
   B. Gingivitis
   C. Mucositis
   D. Dysgeusia

3. Identify the specific interventions that should be addressed before cancer therapy.

   _____   _____

   _____   _____

   _____

4. All of the following oral structures are classified as cancers of the head and neck. Identify the structures that are considered to be true oral cancers.

   1) Lips   4) Retromolar areas

   2) Brain   5) Hard and soft palate

   3) Eyes   6) Thyroid

5. List the three ways the Tumor, Node, Metastasis (TNM) System categorizes the stages and progression of tumors.

1) T = _____

2) N = _____

3) M = _____

6. Explain the dental hygienist's role after a patient has completed head and neck cancer therapy.

_____

_____

_____

_____

_____

_____

_____

_____

_____

7. Which term defines the movement of malignant cells into blood or lymphatic tissue as well as the spread into other regions?
A. Cancer
B. Metastasis
C. Oral squamous cell carcinoma
D. Tumor

8. List the four components of the concept of field cancerization (cancer fields).

1) _____

2) _____

3) _____

4) _____

Learning Activities

1. Discuss some of the benefits to a patient who is part of a multidisciplinary team approach to cancer treatment.

_____

_____

_____

_____

_____

_____

_____

_____

_____

_____

2. Name the most common cancers in the United States.

_____

_____

_____

_____

_____

_____

_____

_____

_____

_____

3. Consider a patient undergoing chemotherapy; discuss the role of the dental hygienist as related to treatment planning within the interdisciplinary care.

_____

_____

_____

_____

_____

_____

_____

_____

_____

_____

_____

4. Discuss the acute symptoms that can result from chemotherapy and radiation therapy.

_____

_____

_____

_____

_____

_____

_____

_____

_____

_____

Board Style Review Questions

1. Match the staging classification with the corresponding definition.

   _____ Stage I   A. Extensive, beyond the regional site, across several tissue layers

   _____ Stage II   B. Localized, defined to site of origin

   _____ Stage III   C. Widely dispersed

   _____ Stage IV   D. Regional, in nearby structures

2. All of the following interventions should be completed before cancer therapy *except* for one. Which of the following procedures is the *exception?*
   A. All carious teeth should be restored.
   B. All teeth with a poor prognosis should be extracted at least 2 days before radiation therapy is started.
   C. Nonsurgical periodontal therapy.
   D. Provision of education to cover possible oral complications associated with treatment.

3. Treatment of oral candidiasis includes which of the following:
   1) Zinc sulfate supplements
   2) Nystatin
   3) Clotrimazole
   4) Omeprazole
       A. 1 and 2
       B. 1 and 3
       C. 2 and 3
       D. 3 and 4

4. The management of xerostomia to reduce risk of radiation caries should include which of the following recommendations?
   A. Use of salivary substitutes
   B. Professionally applied fluoride
   C. Use of casein phophopeptide with amorphous calcium phosphate
   D. None of these
   E. All of the above

5. All of the following statements are true of oral squamous cell carcinoma (OSCC) *except* for one. Which one is the *exception?*
   A. OSCC originates from oral keratinocytes where DNA mutations can be spontaneous.
   B. OSCC is derived from epithelium.
   C. More than 90% of head and neck cancers are oral squamous cell carcinoma.
   D. The epithelium of the scalp, skin, and muscle is affected.

6. Which types of cells do not invade tissues or travel to distant sites?
   A. Benign cells
   B. Dysplastic cells
   C. Malignant cells
   D. Metastatic cells

7. Patients undergoing chemotherapy usually experience acute complications that heal after treatment ends. Patients receiving direct radiation therapy to the head and neck region may have extended or chronic complications.
   A. Both statements are true.
   B. The first statement is true; the second is false.
   C. Both statements are false.
   D. The first statement is false; the second is true.

8. The risk of oral cancer is inversely correlated to the degree of tobacco exposure; therefore, it is important in clinical care to calculate a pack year for your patient.
   A. The statement and the reason are both correct.
   B. The statement is correct; the reason is incorrect.
   C. The statement and the reason are both incorrect.
   D. The statement is incorrect; the reason is correct.

9. Your patient has smoked one-half a pack of cigarettes every day for the last 20 years. Calculate this patient's pack year and select the correct choice.
   A. Number of pack years = 10
   B. Number of pack years = 20
   C. Number of pack years = 50
   D. Number of pack years = 100
   E. Number of pack years = 200

10. Incidence rates of cancer in the United States are higher in men than in women. Approximately one in three women in the United States will develop cancer in her lifetime.
    A. Both statements are correct
    B. The first statement is correct; the second is incorrect.
    C. Both statements are incorrect.
    D. The first statement is incorrect; the second statement is correct

REFERENCES

1. Cancer facts & figures. Atlanta. GA: American Cancer Society. http://www.cancer.org/research/cancerfactsfigures/cancerfactsfigures/cancer-facts-figures-2012. Updated 2012. Accessed October 3, 2015.
2. Taylor C, Munro AJ, Glynne-Jones R, et al. Multidisciplinary team working in cancer: what is the evidence? *BMJ.* 2010;340:c951.

Rubrics/Process Evaluations

Process Evaluation Template

Cancer Risk Assessment

Evaluation Criteria	Criteria Met? (Y/N)	Comments
Thorough head and neck examination.		
Thorough review of history of alcohol use.		
Thorough review of history of tobacco use.		
Pack year calculated if applicable.		
Education provided to patient on cancer incidence.		
Risk factors reviewed and explained to patient.		
Education about the signs and symptoms of cancer.		
Instruction provided to patient as to how to perform a self-examination.		
Tobacco cessation education, resources provided.		
Documentation appropriately noted in treatment notes.		
Referral provided if necessary.		

Chapter 46 | Pediatric Patient

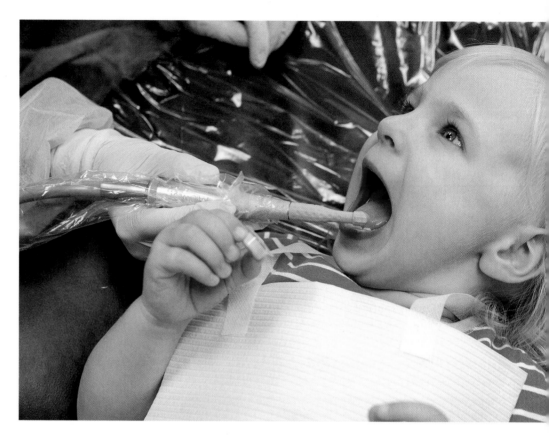

LEARNING OBJECTIVES

After reading this chapter, the student should be able to:

46.1 Discuss the importance of positive dental experiences for the pediatric patient as they relate to achieving a lifetime of good oral health.

46.2 Outline the differences between the surgical model and the medical model approach to oral health.

46.3 Provide appropriate anticipatory guidance to a child's parent or caregiver.

46.4 List several methods to positively engage or develop rapport with the pediatric patient.

46.5 Define the term *dental home* and its significance to oral health.

KEY CONCEPTS

• There has been a paradigm shift in pediatric dentistry from a surgical model to a medical/preventive approach.

• A lifetime of oral health begins before birth.

• Oral-care plans are tailored to each patient's needs and abilities.

• Anticipatory guidance is a part of every child's dental visit.

• Communication with the child's parent or caregiver is essential at every visit.

RELEVANCE TO CLINICAL PRACTICE

The goal of dentistry is the health and preservation of the human dentition—a lifetime of oral health. The child's potential to achieve a lifetime of oral health is largely dependent on the environment he or she lives in and the guidance and manner in which dental care is provided. Understanding and utilizing the knowledge gained in this chapter will allow the dental hygienist to deliver preventive services that are appropriate and cultivate successful oral health behaviors over the child's lifetime.

The Basics

1. The American Dental Association (ADA) recommends that children be scheduled for an initial dental evaluation:
   A. Within 3 months of eruption of the first tooth
   B. Within 6 months of eruption of the first tooth
   C. When they are 2 to 3 years old
   D. After 1-year-old when the child can sit alone in the dental chair.

2. At what age is eruption of the primary teeth generally complete?
   A. 0 to 12 months
   B. 12 to 24 months
   C. 24 to 36 months
   D. 36 to 48 months

3. List the non-nutritive habits.

   1) _____
   2) _____
   3) _____
   4) _____
   5) _____
   6) _____

4. Provide examples of developmental changes that the hygienist should acknowledge at appointments.

   1)   4)

   2)   5)

   3)

5. A mother's health does not affect the development of the primary dentition. However, a mother's use of medication such as tetracycline can affect the developing primary dentition.
   A. Both statements are true.
   B. The first statement is true; the second statement is false.
   C. Both statements are false.
   D. The first statement is false; the second statement is true.

6. The transitional phase is signified by exfoliation of the:
   A. Mandibular central incisors
   B. Mandibular lateral incisors
   C. Maxillary central incisors
   D. Maxillary lateral incisors

7. Enamel formation is complete by 3 years. Root development is complete by 1 year.
   A. Both statements are true.
   B. The first statement is true; the second is false.
   C. Both statements are false.
   D. The first statement is false; the second statement is true.

8. Eruption of the first permanent teeth, the mandibular first molar, occurs ~ 6 to 7 years. At approximately what age is root development complete?
   A. 10 to 11 years
   B. 11 to 12 years
   C. 12 to 13 years
   D. 14 to 15 years

Learning Activities

1. Before dismissing the patient from the chair, it is beneficial to review the findings of the appointment. The dental hygienist can emphasize the child's strengths, encourage his efforts, and express his belief in his capabilities. Imagine you are dismissing your pediatric patient. Prepare a skit/role-play to demonstrate how you would incorporate this in the clinic.

2. A positive dental experience for the pediatric patient can influence a lifetime of good oral health. Explore the American Dental Hygienists' Association (ADHA) and the American Academy of Pediatric Dentistry (AAPD) websites to locate resources and information on how to create a positive visit for your patient.

3. Create a checklist of ways in which the dental hygienist can develop rapport with the pediatric patient.

Board Style Review Questions

1. The hygienist's approach to patient care will change to accommodate the child's:
   A. Emotional level
   B. Maturity level
   C. Physical level

2. The primary dentition begins to develop in utero at how many weeks of gestation?
   A. 4th week
   B. 7th week
   C. 10th week
   D. 12th week

3. Choose the primary intention of the dental home.
   A. To discuss proper oral hygiene
   B. To monitor speech and language development
   C. To improve access to care
   D. To review non-nutritive habits

4. Dental caries results from tooth-adherent specific bacteria, such as *Streptococcus mutans*. Dental caries is a vertically transmitted disease from caregiver to child.
   A. Both statements are correct.
   B. The first statement is correct; the second statement is incorrect.
   C. Both statements are incorrect.
   D. The first statement is incorrect; the second statement is correct.

5. All of the following are descriptors of the knee-to-knee position *except* for one. Which one is the *exception?*
   A. Allow the child to rest in the lap of the parent.
   B. Provides stabilization of the child.
   C. The child can rest in the dental chair.
   D. It can provide good visualization of the oral cavity by both the parents and providers.

6. Appropriate discussion and counseling should be a part of each pediatric patient's dental visit. Failure to appropriately educate caregivers can lead to dental disease.
   A. Both statements are correct.
   B. The first statement is correct; the second statement is incorrect.
   C. Both statements are incorrect.
   D. The first statement is incorrect; the second statement is correct.

7. A medical model approach supports the idea of prevention of dental diseases. A surgical model involves treating the problem.
   A. Both statements are true.
   B. The first statement is true; the second statement is false.
   C. Both statements are false.
   D. The first statement is false; the second statement is true.

8. The "tell-show-do" technique is categorized as which type of behavior guidance technique?
   A. Desensitization
   B. Distraction
   C. Positive reinforcement
   D. Voice control

9. Which statement best describes baby bottle decay or early childhood caries (ECC)?
   A. The presence of 4 or more decayed, missing, or restored primary teeth.
   B. The presence of 3 or more decayed, missing, or restored primary teeth.
   C. The presence of 2 or more decayed, missing, or restored primary teeth.
   D. The presence of 1 or more decayed, missing, or restored primary teeth.

10. Enamel formation in the permanent dentition is completed by what age?
    A. 7 to 8 years
    B. 8 to 9 years
    C. 9 to 10 years
    D. 10 to 11 years

Rubrics/Process Evaluations

Process Evaluation Template

Dental Hygiene Care for the Pediatric Patient

Evaluation Criteria	Criteria Met? (Y/N)	Comments
Ages 6–12 months The student:		
Completes clinical oral assessment.		
Provides oral counseling for caregivers.		
Removes supra- and subgingival stains and deposits.		
Assesses child's systemic and topical fluoride status.		
Assesses feeding practices (bottle vs. breastfeeding).		
Provides dietary counseling related to oral health.		
Provides age-appropriate injury prevention counseling for orofacial trauma.		
Provides counseling for nonnutritive oral habits (digit, pacifier).		
Provides necessary referrals.		
Completes caries risk assessment.		
Determines appropriate interval for reevaluation.		

Chapter 47 | Men's and Women's Health Issues

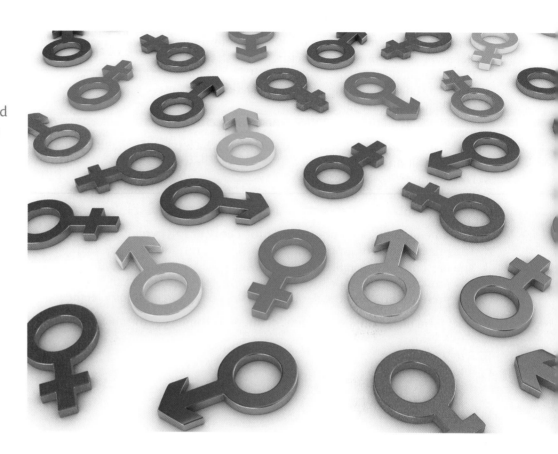

LEARNING OBJECTIVES

After reading this chapter, the student should be able to:

47.1 Define the terms *sex* and *gender*, and explain how they are different.

47.2 Discuss dental hygiene care plan treatment alterations or precautions to be taken during pregnancy.

47.3 Discuss the incidence, risk factors, therapies, and oral complications unique to bisphosphonate-related osteonecrosis of the jaw and osteoradionecrosis.

47.4 Discuss dental hygiene care plan treatment alterations or precautions to be taken with patients with prostate cancer.

47.5 Identify the common signs and symptoms of domestic abuse.

KEY CONCEPTS

- Insight into men's and women's health issues is vital for health-care professionals to understand which issues require consideration of precautions in dental hygiene care.

- Dental hygiene care of patients with prostate cancer requires individualized consideration of systemic and oral complications.

- Risk factors for bisphosphonate-related osteonecrosis of the jaw and osteoradionecrosis include use of IV bisphosphonates, oral bisphosphonates to a lesser degree than IV, patients with or at risk for osteoporosis, and

previous radiation therapy, all of which require consideration of precautions in dental hygiene care.
- Although periodontal therapy has been shown to be safe and leads to improved periodontal conditions in pregnant women, case-related periodontal therapy, with or without systemic antibiotics, does not reduce overall rates of preterm birth and low birth weight.
- Regarding domestic violence, 75% of the physical injuries are to the head, neck, and/or mouth.

RELEVANCE TO CLINICAL PRACTICE

Good oral health involves prevention of disease, in both male and female individuals. It is vital to overall health and well-being at all stages of life. Poor oral health has been linked to heart disease, diabetes, oral cancer, and preterm delivery. Common oral diseases include tooth decay and periodontal diseases, which are caused by bacterial infections. These infections cause an immune response that destroys the gingival tissue and bone that surround the teeth in periodontal disease and, in combination with other factors, cause tooth decay. Dental hygienists should be prepared to understand men's and women's general patterns of growth and development to provide dental hygiene care. Many of the concepts discussed in this chapter will allow the dental hygienist to approach the patient's needs specific to his or her sex and gender, and apply dental hygiene therapies to maintain and improve oral health.

The Basics

1. Sex differences in medicine include sex-specific diseases. They can be described as:
   A. Diseases that occur only in people of one sex.
   B. Diseases more common to one sex.
   C. Diseases that manifest differently.

2. Levels of *B. intermedius* significantly increase during:
   A. Adolescence
   B. Prepuberty
   C. Pregnancy
   D. Puberty

3. The use of oral contraceptives and hormone replacement therapy has been associated with a higher prevalence of:
   A. Temporomandibular disorders (TMD)
   B. Recurrent pain disorders
   C. Sex hormones
   D. Periodontal disease

4. Which drugs are used to treat prostate enlargement?
   1) Alpha-blockers
   2) Beta blockers
   3) Calcium channel blockers
   4) 5-alpha-reductase inhibitors
      A. 1 and 2
      B. 1 and 4
      C. 2 and 3
      D. 3 and 4

5. All of the following hormones affect the microvasculature during pregnancy *except* for one. Which one is the *exception?*
   A. Chronic gonadotropin
   B. Estrogen
   C. Progesterone
   D. Thyroid stimulating hormone

6. What are the symptoms of bisphosphonate-related osteonecrosis of the jaw (BRONJ)?

   _____

   _____

7. Oral health professionals should be familiar with the risks and benefits for pregnant or breastfeeding patients. List the five types of medication that should be carefully considered if prescribed to pregnant or breastfeeding patients.

   1. _____

   2. _____

   3. _____

   4. _____

   5. _____

8. Epulis gravidarum is also referred to as a pregnancy granuloma. Which of these descriptors is incorrect?
   A. It is painless.
   B. It is greater than 2 mm in diameter.
   C. It can occur in healthy women.
   D. It is often the result of poor oral hygiene.

9. Select the appropriate management guidelines for platelet counts less than 30,000/mm³.
   A. No additional support is needed.
   B. Prophylactic antibiotic is recommended.
   C. Platelets should be transfused 1 hour before procedure.
   D. Platelet transfusions are optional for noninvasive treatment.

10. Why is it important to take into account the sex of a person before treatment?

    _____

    _____

Learning Activities

1. With a student partner, practice explaining what is thought to contribute to the increase in gingivitis in pregnant patients.

2. Discuss the risk factors for BRONJ development in small groups.

3. Support the use of bisphosphonates to stop bone loss. Submit a keynote.

4. Describe how the dental hygienist can reduce the risk of supine hypotension syndrome during the treatment of pregnant women. In the clinic, demonstrate how the pregnant woman should be positioned for dental hygiene treatment.

5. Make a checklist of the pretreatment interventions for a patient receiving chemotherapy for prostate cancer.

Board Style Review Questions

1. Eating disorders and trauma are more prevalent among females than males. Smoking is more prevalent among adolescent males.
   A. Both statements are true.
   B. The first statement is true; the second statement is false.
   C. Both statements are false.
   D. The first statement is false; the second statement is true.

2. All of the following determine biological sex at birth *except* for one. Which one is the *exception?*
   A. Presence or absence of a Y chromosome
   B. Internal reproductive anatomy
   C. Presence or absence of an X chromosome
   D. External genitalia

3. Select the term for socially defined differences between men and women.
   A. Gender
   B. Interconceptual
   C. Sex
   D. Sex difference

4. Decreased bone calcification is termed:
   A. Osteonecrosis
   B. Osteopenia
   C. Osteoporosis
   D. Osteoradionecrosis

5. In domestic violence cases, what percentage of physical injuries occurs to the head, neck, and/or mouth?
   A. 10%
   B. 25%
   C. 50%
   D. 75%

6. What are the possible adverse events that can arise from drugs used to treat benign prostatic hyperplasia (BPH)?
   A. Atrial fibrillation
   B. Dizziness or hypotension
   C. Hypertension
   D. Tachycardia

7. Identify the values that the dental hygienist should know before providing treatment to a patient receiving chemotherapy for prostate cancer.
   A. Hemoglobin and platelet count
   B. White blood cell and red blood cell counts
   C. White blood cell count, red blood cell count, and hemoglobin
   D. White blood cell, red blood cell, and platelet counts

8. Intersex is defined as:
   A. A person's gender
   B. A person's self-perceived gender
   C. A group of conditions where there is a discrepancy between the external genitals and the internal genitals
   D. Presence or absence of a Y chromosome

9. Identify the *incorrect* statement.
   A. During puberty, females experience an increased level of sex hormones, which causes a decrease in blood supply to the gingiva.
   B. Females usually experience puberty between 11 and 14 years old.
   C. Males typically experience puberty between 13 and 16 years old.
   D. Puberty is a developmental stage when an individual is capable of reproduction.

10. Bisphosphonates prevent the loss of bone mass. Antiresorptive medications increase the rate of bone formation.
    A. Both statements are correct.
    B. The first statement is correct; the second statement is incorrect.
    C. Both statements are incorrect.
    D. The first statement is incorrect; the second statement is correct.

Chapter 48 | The Elderly

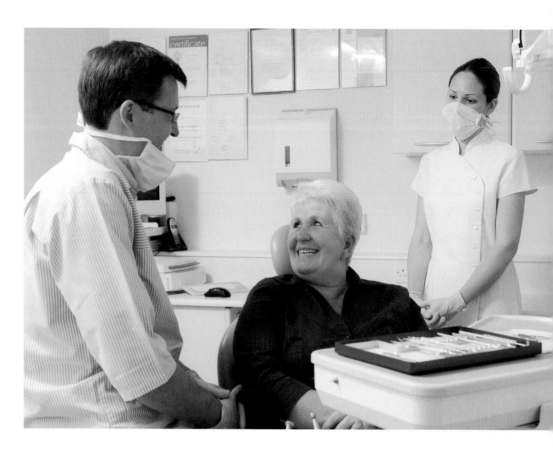

LEARNING OBJECTIVES

After reading this chapter, the student should be able to:

48.1 Identify demographic changes over the past century in American society and discuss how these changes impact current and future oral health-care needs of an aging society.

48.2 Explain the difference between chronological age and functional age.

48.3 Discuss pathophysiological changes associated with age, as well as age-related conditions and systemic diseases common to the elderly.

48.4 Differentiate between normal aging and pathophysiological oral conditions of the elderly.

48.5 Discuss the importance of assessment of the elderly dental patient for treatment planning, patient management, dental hygiene care, and maintenance of oral health.

48.6 Discuss educational and preventive oral health considerations for the elderly patient.

KEY CONCEPTS

• Demographic data project substantial increases in all age brackets of older populations aged 65 and older.

• In older adults, a disparity between a person's chronological age and functional age is common.

- Many older adults require multiple medications for a variety of diseases, challenging both overall health and oral health.
- The dental professional needs to understand both medical and dental complexities of older adults, as well as how complex conditions such as diabetes, multiple medications, and self-care limitations impact oral health and oral care.
- Older adult patients have an increased incidence and prevalence of root caries because of underlying risk factors such as xerostomia.
- When treating older adult patients, dental professionals should focus on prevention rather than restorative care.

RELEVANCE TO CLINICAL PRACTICE

During the past century, the United States has witnessed advancements in both medicine and dentistry, allowing people to live longer and keep their teeth for a lifetime. Vaccines, antibiotics, improved nutrition, and healthier lifestyle practices have helped to increase life expectancy. In addition, systemic and topical fluorides, advanced dental procedures, and better oral hygiene self-care have decreased tooth loss and lowered the edentulous rate. Although these improvements have made significant contributions to the overall health of the U.S. population, they have also introduced a new set of problems caused by a rapidly growing number of aging Americans that have placed increased demands on the medical and dental health-care system in the United States.[1]

The Basics

1. The consumption of grapefruit can increase the absorption of which of the following medications?
   A. Azithromycin
   B. Phenytoin
   C. Simvastatin
   D. Sulfamethoxazole

2. A high-risk drug interaction can occur between angiotensin-converting enzyme (ACE) inhibitors and:
   A. Macrolides
   B. Potassium supplements
   C. Sulfa drugs
   D. Tetracyclines

3. Achlorhydria is an insufficient production of gastric acid in the stomach that affects the gastrointestinal system with aging. This condition decreases the absorption of important nutrients, ultimately putting a person at risk for nutritional deficiencies.
   A. Both statements are correct.
   B. The first statement is correct; the second is incorrect.
   C. Both statements are incorrect.
   D. The first statement is incorrect; the second statement is correct.

4. List three risk factors that impact a person's biological age that can be modified.

1) _____

2) _____

3) _____

5. In the dentition of older adults, what causes a reduction in tooth sensitivity?
   A. Thermal properties increase affecting the patient's perception of pain.
   B. The blood vessels entering the pulp chamber increase.
   C. Osmotic properties increase affecting the patient's perception of pain.
   D. The blood vessels entering the pulp chamber decrease.

6. How old is a person who is considered "older-old"?
   A. Ages 55 to 65
   B. Ages 65 to 75
   C. Ages 75 to 85
   D. Ages 85+

7. Functional age describes how a person's body ages physiologically. The functionally dependent older adult can no longer survive without direct and daily help from others.
   A. Both statements are true.
   B. Both statements are false.
   C. The first statement is true; the second statement is false.
   D. The first statement is false; the second statement is true.

8. People age 60 years and older have the highest incidence of oral cancer. List three risk factors for oral cancer.

1) _____

2) _____

3) _____

9. All of the following drugs can interfere with warfarin (Coumadin) *except* for one. Which of these is the *exception?*
   A. Ciprofloxacin
   B. Clarithromycin
   C. Naproxen
   D. Phenytoin

Learning Activities

1. Differentiate between the functional age groups as related to the activities of daily living (ADLs).

_____

_____

_____

_____

_____

_____

_____

_____

_____

_____

_____

_____

2. In a small group, discuss some of the theories that exist on how the aging process occurs.

_____

_____

_____

_____

_____

_____

_____

_____

_____

_____

_____

_____

Board Style Review Questions

1. The term for increased thirst associated with diabetes is:
   A. Polydipsia
   B. Polyuria
   C. Polyphagia
   D. Polycythemia

2. Which of the following international normalized ratio (INR) ranges is considered safe to perform both noninvasive and invasive dental procedures?
   A. ≥3.5
   B. 3.0 to 3.4
   C. 2.5 to 3.0
   D. 2.0 to 2.5

3. After a transient ischemic attack or stroke, elective and invasive dental care should be deferred for how long following the event?
   A. There is no required deferment period
   B. 6 mo
   C. 1 mo
   D. 3 mo

4. Which of the four taste perceptions declines in older adults?
   A. Salty
   B. Sweet
   C. Bitter
   D. Sour

5. INR measures the time it takes for a patient's blood to clot. An INR of 3.5 may indicate that the blood is clotting too fast.
   A. Both statements are correct.
   B. The first statement is correct; the second statement is incorrect.
   C. Both statements are incorrect.
   D. The first statement is incorrect; the second statement is correct.

6. In aging adults, bone mass decrease occurs when:
   A. Osteoblasts stay the same; osteoclasts decrease.
   B. Osteoblasts decrease; osteoclasts decrease.
   C. Osteoblasts decrease; osteoclasts stay the same.
   D. Osteoblasts increase; osteoclasts increase.

7. Xerostomia is a normal part of aging; therefore, noticeable changes in the amount and flow of saliva can be expected as a healthy person ages.
   A. Both the statement and the reason are correct.
   B. The statement is incorrect; the reason is correct.
   C. Both the statement and the reason are incorrect.
   D. The statement is correct; the reason is incorrect.

8. The dental hygienist should refer a patient for a definitive diagnosis if a lesion persists for more than:
   A. 2 weeks
   B. 2 mo
   C. 3 mo
   D. 6 mo

9. Oral cancer can occur in any part of the oral cavity, however, it *most* frequently appears on which of the following structures?
   1) Oral pharynx
   2) Lateral borders of the tongue
   3) Buccal mucosa
   4) Floor of the mouth
   5) Lips
      A. 1 and 4
      B. 2 and 3
      C. 1, 4, and 5
      D. 2, 4, and 5

10. The term for increased appetite associated with diabetes is:
    A. Polydipsia
    B. Polyphagia
    C. Polyuria
    D. Polycythemia

REFERENCES

1. U.S. Department of Health and Human Services. *Oral Health in America: A Report of the Surgeon General—Executive Summary.* Rockville, MD: U.S. Department of Health and Human Services, National Institute of Dental and Craniofacial Research, National Institutes of Health; 2000.

Rubrics/Process Evaluations

Process Evaluation Template		
Physiological Changes Review		
Evaluation Criteria	**Criteria Met? (Y/N)**	**Comments**
(Student will interview an elderly patient to identify physiological changes affecting each of the body systems noted below.)		
Cardiovascular: Student discusses potential symptoms especially hypotension with the patient.		
Respiratory: Student reviews potential respiratory concerns (diminished breathing after physical activity).		
Gastrointestinal: Student notes symptoms of potential nutrient deficiency (tingling in arms, legs, fatigue, dementia).		
Urinary: Symptoms associated with dehydration are noted (sleepiness, irritability, delirium), excessive/infrequent urination.		
Endocrine: Student asks about altered functions, such as body temperature, stress response, heart function, response to insulin.		
Brain and nervous system: Student reviews for inability to stay focused, difficulty combining words, short-term memory loss, slower reaction time.		
Immune system: Student identifies changes in immune system to allow for early intervention/modification to treatment.		
Musculoskeletal system: Student notes loss of height, gait problems.		
Sensory system (hearing): Student records symptoms of presbycusis and tinnitus.		
Sensory system (vision): Student records difficulty seeing at close range, reading small print.		
Integumentary system: Student reviews for skin infections, altered body temperature.		
Patient interview conducted in an appropriate setting. Patient seated upright and at eye level to student.		

Chapter 49 | Physical Impairment

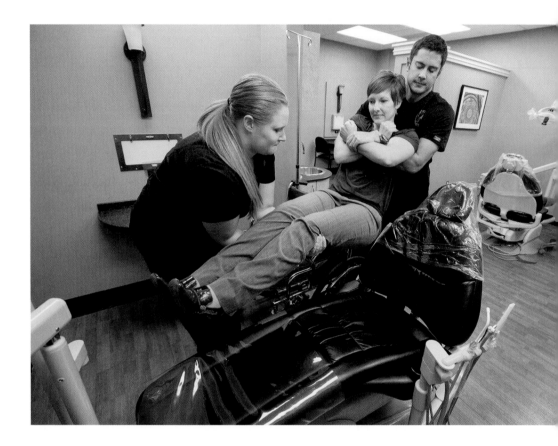

LEARNING OBJECTIVES

After reading this chapter, the student should be able to:

49.1 Identify barriers for people with physical impairments.

49.2 Describe the causes and age of onset of common physical impairments.

49.3 List various physical conditions of people with physical impairments.

49.4 Describe the clinical considerations for treatment for people with physical impairments.

49.5 Describe treatment modalities and adaptations for people with physical impairments.

49.6 Describe modifications that the dental hygienist may make when providing care to people with physical impairments.

49.7 Describe the conditions, causes, and incidence of various impairments.

49.8 Perform a two-person wheelchair transfer.

KEY CONCEPTS

- Lack of access to dental care is a critical problem for people with physical impairments.
- Maintaining good oral health is particularly important for the overall health of people with physical impairments.

• Successful provision of oral hygiene care for people with physical impairments requires a basic general knowledge of conditions resulting in degrees of impairment.

RELEVANCE TO CLINICAL PRACTICE

With an increasingly older population and medical advances, the prevalence of people with physical impairments is increasing. Chronic disabling diseases affect millions of Americans and compromise oral health and functioning. Those who seek care may be faced with health practitioners who lack the training and cultural competence to communicate effectively to provide needed services.[1] The dental hygienist must have the knowledge and ability to effectively serve people with physical impairments.

The Basics

1. Your patient is used to being transferred from her wheelchair by her care provider. Therefore, you should perform a single-person transfer from the wheelchair to the dental chair.
   A. Both the statement and the reason are correct.
   B. The statement is correct; the reason is incorrect.
   C. Both the statement and the reason are incorrect.
   D. The statement is incorrect; the reason is correct.

2. Persons with physical impairments commonly take antiseizure drugs. All of the following are antiseizure drugs *except* for one. Which one is the *exception?*
   A. Atropine
   B. Dilantin
   C. Depakote
   D. Phenobarbital
   E. Tegretol

3. Which of these is considered one of the basic activities of daily living (BADL)?
   A. Using the telephone
   B. Preparing a meal
   C. Grooming
   D. Using public transportation

4. Oral hygiene instruction can be simplified by using the "tell-show-do" approach. Recall the steps to this approach.

   1) _____   4) _____

   2) _____   5) _____

   3) _____

5. Select the statement that best describes normalization.
   A. Inclusion of persons with impairments in societal activities.
   B. Training impaired individuals to lead more independent lives.
   C. Focus on a person's abilities not impairments.

6. List the oral characteristics that are more common to persons with physical impairments compared with the general population.

   1) _____   4) _____

   2) _____   5) _____

   3) _____   6) _____

7. Rings of bone called vertebrae surround the spinal cord. In general, the lower the spinal injury occurs, the more dysfunction a person will experience.
   A. Both statements are true.
   B. Both statements are false.
   C. The first statement is true; the second statement is false.
   D. The first statement is false; the second statement is true.

8. Latex allergy is prevalent among people with which of these conditions?
   A. Cystic fibrosis
   B. Muscular dystrophy
   C. Spina bifida
   D. Spinal muscular atrophy

9. Which of these is the most common degenerative disease of the nervous system in children?
   A. Cystic fibrosis
   B. Muscular dystrophy
   C. Spina bifida
   D. Spinal muscular atrophy

10. In a two-person wheelchair transfer, the first clinician should place his/her arms under the patient's upper arms and grasp the patient's wrists. The second clinician should place both hands under the patient's lower thighs.
    A. Both statements are correct.
    B. The first statement is correct; the second statement is incorrect.
    C. Both statements are incorrect.
    D. The first statement is incorrect; the second statement is correct.

Learning Activities

1. Construct a chart that outlines the physical impairments with the associated barriers, cause, age of onset, and clinical considerations for each.

2. Your patient has a physical impairment and has difficulty moving his toothbrush across his teeth primarily because it is difficult to grasp. What recommendations/modifications would you suggest? Fabricate a brush for this patient and share with your class.

_____

_____

_____

_____

_____

_____

_____

_____

_____

_____

_____

_____

_____

_____

_____

3. Research an adaptive product for patients with physical impairments.

_____

_____

_____

_____

_____

_____

_____

_____

_____

_____

_____

_____

_____

_____

_____

_____

_____

_____

Board Style Review Questions

1. Which of the following is an inherited condition?
    A. Cystic fibrosis
    B. Cerebral palsy
    C. Cleft palate
    D. Meningitis

2. All of the following are autoimmune conditions *except* for one. Which one is the *exception?*
    A. Type 1 diabetes
    B. Rheumatoid arthritis
    C. Bell palsy
    D. Multiple sclerosis

3. Identify the phrase that does not represent "people-first language."
    A. Handicapped parking.
    B. The patient has diabetes.
    C. She receives special needs services.
    D. He is a person with epilepsy.

4. All of the following demonstrate appropriate wheelchair etiquette *except* for one. Which one is the *exception?*
   A. Do not automatically push the wheelchair for the patient.
   B. Treatment should always be provided in the wheelchair so it is more comfortable for the patient.
   C. Do not lean on a patient's wheelchair.
   D. Adjust your position (kneel, sit down, squat) to share eye level with the patient if the conversation lasts more than a few minutes.

5. If you are uncertain about how to interact with a person who has a disability, you should assume that the person needs help. You should accept that a disability exists.
   A. Both statements are correct.
   B. The first statement is correct; the second statement is incorrect.
   C. Both statements are incorrect.
   D. The first statement is incorrect; the second statement is correct.

6. A genetic disease characterized by progressive weakness and degeneration of the skeletal muscles describes which of these conditions?
   A. A traumatic brain injury
   B. Quadriplegia
   C. Paraplegia
   D. Muscular dystrophy

7. There are many barriers to access to health care especially for those people with impairments. Select the primary obstacle for people with impairments as related to health care.
   A. Architectural barriers
   B. Financial barriers
   C. Transportation barriers
   D. Attitudinal barriers

8. Which of these types of muscular dystrophy primarily affects boys?
   A. Duchenne
   B. Facioscapulohumeral
   C. Myotonic
   D. Cystic fibrosis

9. Cleft palate is considered:
   A. An inherited condition
   B. An acquired condition
   C. A developmental condition
   D. A congenital condition

10. Which of these conditions is an autosomal recessive hereditary disease characterized by progressive hypotonia and muscular weakness?
   A. Spina bifida
   B. Muscular dystrophy
   C. Spinal muscular atrophy
   D. Cystic fibrosis

REFERENCES

1. Altman B, Bernstein A. *Disability and health in the United States, 2001–2005*. Hyattsville, MD: National Center for Health Statistics; 2008.

Rubrics/Process Evaluations

Process Evaluation Template

Transfer from Dental Chair to Wheelchair

Evaluation Criteria	Criteria Met? (Y/N)	Comments
Student positions the wheelchair close and parallel to the dental chair.		
Student locks the wheels in place, turns the castors forward, and removes the armrest on the wheelchair.		
Student raises the dental chair until slightly higher than the wheelchair and removes dental chair armrest.		
Student transfers any special padding.		
Patient is transferred using the two-person transfer technique.		
Student repositions the patient in the wheelchair.		
Student attaches the safety belt (if present).		
Student replaces the armrests and foot rests.		

Chapter 50 | Alternative Practice Settings

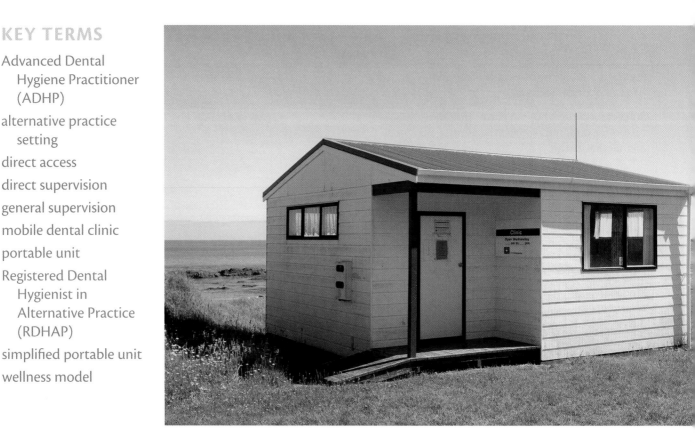

LEARNING OBJECTIVES

After reading this chapter, the student should be able to:

50.1 Define the issues in access to oral health prevention measures and care.

50.2 Identify venues beyond the traditional office setting where dental hygienists provide access to care.

50.3 Describe alternative setting methods and identify resources for delineating state laws related to those settings.

50.4 List the equipment necessary to facilitate delivery of care in alternative practice settings.

50.5 Identify the roles dental hygienists play in alternative settings.

50.6 Discuss the protocols and techniques for delivering care in alternative settings.

KEY CONCEPTS

- Access to a Registered Dental Hygienist is vital to clients' overall health, and there are many settings for delivery of care.
- Preventive and operative dental hygiene services can be delivered in a variety of settings by adapting practices to the location and using proper equipment.
- Availability of dental care in alternative settings allows all patients to receive preventive strategies and operative care.

RELEVANCE TO CLINICAL PRACTICE

Many Americans lack access to adequate dental care, resulting in extensive dental disease.[1] Traditional models for increasing access to care expand delivery systems such as private dental offices and community clinics. Newer models that utilize nonoffice settings and expand the role of dental hygienists are proving effective in eliminating many of the obstacles to access to care. In states that allow **direct access,** dental hygienists can "initiate dental treatment based on their assessment of the patient's needs without authorization from a dentist, treat the patient without the presence of a dentist, and maintain a provider-patient relationship."[1] Since 1995, the number of states that allow direct access has increased from 5 to 36.[2]

As the dental profession embraces the **wellness model** of guiding patients toward risk reduction and disease prevention, dental hygienists play a major role in the prevention of disease, from dental caries to aspiration pneumonia. Dental hygienists continue to expand the venues in which they serve and develop methods of service to meet their clients' needs.

The Basics

1. List six barriers to oral health care.

    1) _____

    2) _____

    3) _____

    4) _____

    5) _____

    6) _____

2. Which dental care provider model was proposed by the American Dental Hygienists' Association (ADHA)?
    A. Advanced Dental Hygiene Practitioner (ADHP)
    B. Dental therapist
    C. Registered Dental Hygienist in Alternative Practice (RDHAP)
    D. Wellness model

3. Describe the limitations of mobile dental clinics.

    _____

    _____

4. Choose the *best* descriptor for simplified portable units.
    A. Lightweight, self-contained, and have a compressor for suction.
    B. Use available resources to meet the needs of those who cannot come to the dental office.
    C. Self-contained dental operations with all equipment necessary for delivery of treatment.
    D. Power to deliver complete care but can be quite loud.

5. Explain the benefits of portable dental units.

_____

_____

_____

_____

6. Which type of supervision allows for performance of duties that are based on instructions given by a licensed dentist, but not requiring the physical presence of the supervising dentist during the performance of these procedures?
   A. Authorized supervision
   B. Direct supervision
   C. General supervision
   D. Indirect supervision

7. Explain the benefits and limitations to the backpack model for oral health care.

_____

_____

_____

8. Flying dental hygienists _most_ often provide services to:
   A. Rural areas that have no access to care.
   B. Low income, homeless, those with limited transportation.
   C. Patients in private practice in underserved areas.
   D. Patients who have difficulty leaving their bed or changing positions.

9. The lower the International Normalized Ratio, the longer it takes blood to clot. It takes the average person 1 to 6 minutes to clot.
   A. Both statements are correct.
   B. The first statement is correct; the second statement is incorrect.
   C. Both statements are incorrect.
   D. The first statement is incorrect; the second statement is correct.

10. Which level of the partial thromboplastin time (PTT) signifies a severe bleeding problem?
   A. Less than 50 sec
   B. Greater than 50 sec
   C. 11 to 16 sec
   D. 25 to 40 sec

Learning Activities

1. Identify an area that has a shortage of dental care providers. How could you address this access to care issue?

_____

_____

_____

_____

2. In small groups, discuss the challenges and rewards of being an independent practice dental hygienist.

Board Style Review Questions

1. Choose all that relate to the dental hygiene scope of practice.
   1) General supervision duties that are based on instructions given by a licensed dentist.
   2) Procedures that must be checked and approved by the supervising dentist.
   3) Allowable duties a dental hygienist may perform.
   4) The location where dental hygiene duties may be performed.
      A. 1 and 3
      B. 1 and 4
      C. 2 and 3
      D. 3 and 4

2. Which level of supervision requires the dentist to be present and in some states the procedures to be checked and approved by the supervising dentist before the patient is dismissed?
   A. Direct
   B. Independent
   C. Indirect
   D. General

3. The wellness model allows:
   A. The dental hygienist to independently provide care.
   B. For increased access to care.
   C. The dental professional to guide patients toward risk reduction.
   D. The dental professional to guide patients toward disease reduction.

4. Adapting to alternative practice settings involves all of the following *except* for one. Which one is the *exception?*
   A. Understanding the services that are needed.
   B. Understanding the patients' needs.
   C. Advocating for policy change.
   D. Recognizing the type of equipment that is needed to meet the needs of patients.

5. Mobile dental clinics are:
   1) Self-contained dental operatories on wheels
   2) Lightweight, self-contained, and have a compressor for suction
   3) Limited by the large amount of space they require for setup
   4) Limited by the noise they produce
      A. 1 and 3
      B. 1 and 4
      C. 2 and 3
      D. 2 and 4

6. All of the following are true of direct access *except* for one. Which one is the *exception?*
   A. The dental hygienist can initiate dental treatment based on assessment of the patient's needs.
   B. The dental hygienist can treat the patient without the presence of a dentist.
   C. The dental hygienist needs authorization from a dentist before starting treatment.
   D. The dental hygienist can maintain a provider-patient relationship.

7. Select the unit that is considered a dental office on wheels.
   A. Independent clinics
   B. Mobile dental clinics
   C. Portable units
   D. Simplified portable units

8. Which type of dental unit can generally be plugged directly into a 110 volt outlet?
   A. Independent clinics
   B. Mobile dental clinics
   C. Portable units
   D. Simplified portable units

9. The federal government requires all of the following of skilled nursing facilities *except* for one. Which one is the *exception?*
   A. They must provide each resident with access to dental services.
   B. They must ensure that residents have an oral examination every year.
   C. They must provide daily oral care to the residents.
   D. They must find alternative sources to fund services if the oral health services are not included in the facilities fees and the resident cannot afford to pay for care.

10. Identify the advantage of the dental hygienist practicing in a freestanding building.
    A. The dental hygienist can provide care to those who are bedridden.
    B. School-age children whose parents have limited time off from work are able to receive treatment on the premises.
    C. The dental hygienist can provide care to those who are in a confined setting.
    D. It allows a community to have direct access to care in areas where they are not able to access dental services.

REFERENCES

1. American Dental Hygienists' Association. Advocacy. 2012. Available from: http://www.adha.org/direct-access.
2. American Dental Hygienists' Association. Direct access states. 2013. Available from: http://www.adha.org/resources-docs/7513_Direct_Access_to_Care_from_DH.pdf.

Part X

Emergency Management

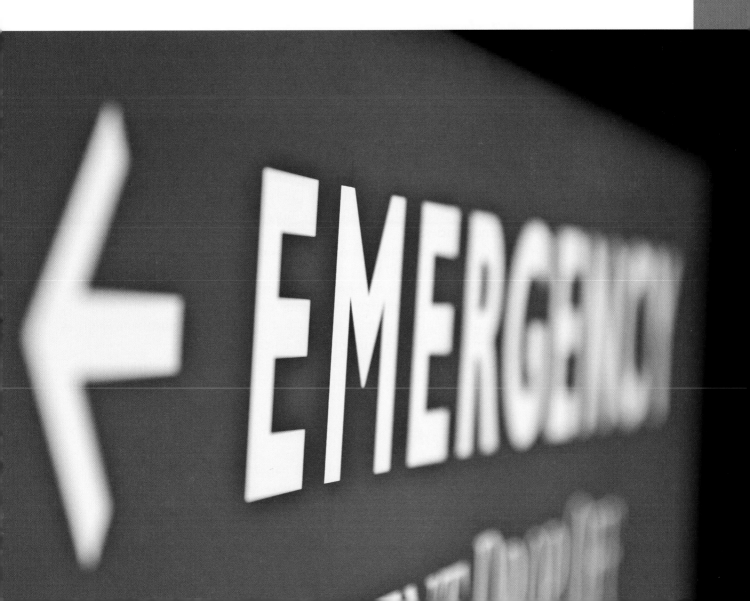

Chapter 51 | Dental and Medical Emergencies

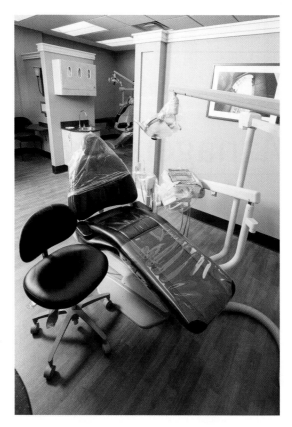

LEARNING OBJECTIVES

After reading this chapter, the student should be able to:

51.1 Identify strategies for reducing the risk of a potential emergency.

51.2 Explain the need for routine training in the management of medical emergencies.

51.3 Determine the patient's American Society of Anesthesiologists Physical Status Classification.

51.4 Recognize signs and symptoms of dental and medical emergencies.

51.5 Develop an emergency management action plan.

51.6 Identify equipment used for the management of medical emergencies.

51.7 Prepare for the prevention of a medical emergency.

51.8 Discuss the management of dental and medical emergencies.

51.9 Explain the role of oral appliances in overall safety and in preventing oral trauma.

KEY CONCEPTS

• Prevention is the first component in managing an emergency.

• Appropriate training and preparation are key aspects of emergency management for all office personnel.

• Recognition and management of emergencies is an element of comprehensive care.

RELEVANCE TO CLINICAL PRACTICE

As a health-care professional, the dental hygienist assumes the responsibility to take the necessary measures needed to prevent or minimize the risk of an emergency occurring during treatment. However, it must be anticipated that an emergency will occur at some point in one's career. It is therefore critical that the dental hygienist be prepared to recognize and manage medical emergencies.

The first component in managing medical emergencies is prevention. It is the hygienist's responsibility to identify potential emergencies. This is accomplished through patient observation and the completion of a comprehensive medical history at each appointment. These steps provide the hygienist with an opportunity to identify those patients who are medically compromised or present with risk factors that may increase the likelihood of an emergency. With this knowledge the hygienist can make appropriate modifications regarding treatment and patient management to reduce the risk of emergencies.

The second component of successful management of medical emergencies is preparedness. All members of the dental team should be aware of their role in the event of an emergency. Accomplishing this includes appropriate and routine training, a clear action plan for dealing with emergencies, and regular review of policies and procedures regarding emergency management.

The Basics

1. In an emergency situation involving a child, rescue breathing should follow which of these guidelines?
   A. 1 breath every 3 to 5 sec
   B. 1 breath every 5 to 6 sec
   C. 1 breath every 6 to 8 sec
   D. 1 breath every 10 to 12 sec

2. What percentage of children will encounter a tooth injury by the time they are adolescents?
   A. 10%
   B. 25%
   C. 50%
   D. 75%

3. How often should a member of the dental team check the equipment and ensure items are not expired?
   A. Weekly
   B. Monthly
   C. Quarterly
   D. Biannually

4. All of the following masks for an oxygen delivery system have a flow rate of 10 to 15 L/min *except* for one. Which one is the *exception?*
   A. Bag-valve mask
   B. Nonrebreather mask
   C. Face mask

5. What medical emergency equipment should all dental offices be equipped with?

1) _____

2) _____

3) _____

4) _____

6. Your patient reports taking levothyroxine and a multivitamin daily. He reports no other systemic conditions. Choose the American Society of Anesthesiologist Physical Status Classification that you would designate for this patient.
   A. ASA PS 1
   B. ASA PS 2
   C. ASA PS 3
   D. ASA PS 4

7. Compression depth for adult CPR is:
   A. 1/2 in.
   B. 1 in.
   C. 1.5 in.
   D. 2 in.

8. List the drugs that the Council of Scientific Affairs recommends for inclusion in an emergency drug kit.

   _____

   _____

   _____

   _____

   _____

   _____

   _____

   _____

9. All of the following are signs of acute fluoride toxicity *except* for one. Which one is the *exception?*
   A. Abdominal pain
   B. Headache
   C. Nausea
   D. Respiratory depression

Learning Activities

1. Practice running an emergency medical action plan.

2. Create a case scenario for management of a medical emergency. Practice the scenario with classmates.

3. Role-play with a classmate. Imagine that your "patient" is an athlete. Explain to him/her the importance of an oral appliance in order to prevent oral trauma.

Board Style Review Questions

1. Match the following descriptors to the appropriate American Society of Anesthesiologists Physical Status classification (ASA PS).

   _____ ASA PS 1   A. Postpone elective dental care

   _____ ASA PS 2   B. Palliative treatment for pain management only

   _____ ASA PS 3   C. Treatment not indicated

   _____ ASA PS 4   D. No modifications indicated

   _____ ASA PS 5   E. Exercise caution during treatment

   _____ ASA PS 6   F. Medical consultation when indicated

2. An "E"/M-24 oxygen cylinder provides how many minutes of oxygen?
   A. 15 min
   B. 30 min
   C. 1 hr
   D. 1 to 2 hr

3. Select the appropriate treatment for a nosebleed.
   1) Place the patient in the upright position.
   2) Place the patient in the supine position.
   3) Have the patient lean forward.
   4) Have the patient lean backward.
      A. 1 and 2
      B. 1 and 3
      C. 2 and 4
      D. 3 and 4

4. Deep rapid breath, shortness of breath, and tightness in the chest are symptoms of which condition?
   A. Syncope
   B. Shock
   C. Hyperventilation
   D. Insulin reaction

5. Anaphylaxis and an allergic reaction are both responses to an allergen. Administration of epinephrine is always required for both of these emergency situations.
   A. Both statements are correct.
   B. The first statement is correct; the second statement is incorrect.
   C. Both statements are incorrect.
   D. The first statement is incorrect; the second statement is correct.

6. Which of the following inhaled emergency drugs is used to treat syncope?
   A. Albuterol
   B. Aromatic ammonia
   C. Bronchodilator
   D. Oxygen

7. Oxygen is the most useful drug in an emergency. It is indicated in all emergency situations except hyperventilation.
   A. Both statements are true.
   B. The first statement is true; the second statement is false.
   C. Both statements are false.
   D. The first statement is false; the second statement is true.

8. Stressors associated with dental fear or anxiety can increase the risk of acute medical emergencies. Therefore, a thorough psychological assessment is necessary to determine a patient's outlook on dental treatment.
   A. Both the statement and the reason are correct.
   B. The statement is correct; the reason is incorrect.
   C. Both the statement and the reason are incorrect.
   D. The statement is incorrect; the reason is correct.

9. The patient should be placed in the upright position during all of the following medical emergencies *except* for one. Which one is the *exception?*
   A. Angina pectoris
   B. Heart failure
   C. Asthma
   D. Hemorrhage

10. Shock-like symptoms, low blood pressure, and/or weakness are signs and symptoms of which of the following conditions?
    A. Diabetic coma
    B. Angina pectoris
    C. Anaphylaxis
    D. Adrenal crisis

Rubrics/Process Evaluations

Process Evaluation Template		
Medical Emergency Preparedness		
Evaluation Criteria	**Criteria Met? (Y/N)**	**Comments**
Student has completed basic life support training.		
Student has located the posted emergency contact information.		
Student has reviewed the action plan and can recall the process/procedure for a medical emergency.		
Student knows his/her responsibilities during a medical emergency situation.		
Student has located and reviewed the basic first aid kit.		
Student has located and reviewed the emergency drug kit.		
Student has located and reviewed the portable oxygen tanks and accessories.		
Student has located and reviewed the automated external defibrillator (AED).		
Student submits a "mock" emergency treatment report form.		
Student recognizes information that may be requested when reporting an emergency to EMS (911).		

Part XI

Future Vision

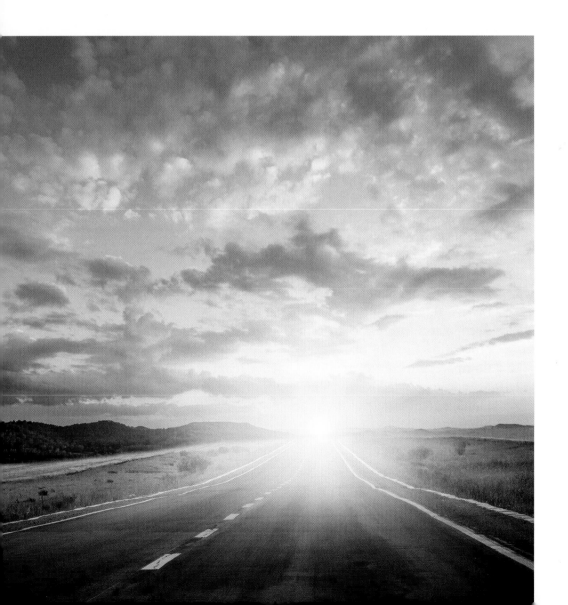

Chapter 52 | Practice Management

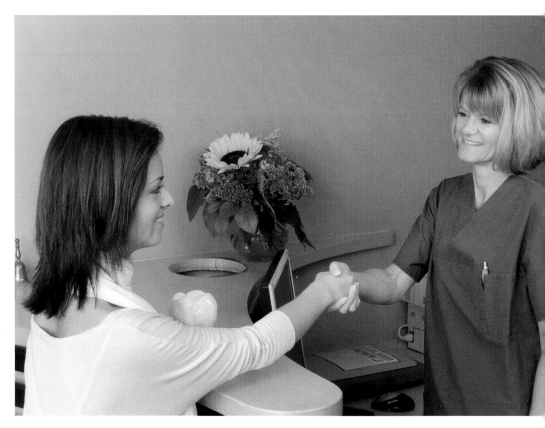

LEARNING OBJECTIVES

After reading this chapter, the student should be able to:

52.1 Define and discuss leadership in the dental practice.

52.2 Discuss components of communication.

52.3 Establish professional and personal goals.

52.4 Develop a practice vision and mission.

52.5 Understand hygiene and office production goals.

52.6 Explain dental benefit information to patients.

52.7 Discuss financial options with patients.

52.8 Recognize appropriate Current Dental Terminology codes for hygiene
    procedures.

52.9 Compare and contrast various practice team meetings.

52.10 Schedule an effective hygiene appointment as it relates to the practice
     management aspect of the practice.

52.11 Summarize habits of highly effective practices.

KEY CONCEPTS

• Leadership within the dental practice is not only the responsibility of the
  dentist/owner, but involves all team members.

- Communication is essential in all areas of the dental practice, between dentist and team members, between team members, and between patient and dentist/team members. Communication influences patient relationships and retention.
- The hygienist and all team members need to understand the vision, mission, and goals of the practice.
- The dental practice is a business that must be run efficiently to survive and prosper.

RELEVANCE TO CLINICAL PRACTICE

Dental hygienists devote most of their time to educating and motivating patients, and practicing their clinical skills. Despite its clinical focus, however, dentistry is a business, and hygienists need to develop leadership, communication, and problem-solving skills to be successful. Knowledge of and proficiency in using efficient business and clinical management systems are also necessary to contribute to the dental practice's success.

The Basics

1. Accounts receivable are the amounts due to the practice. These accounts are solely from insurance balances.
   A. Both statements are correct.
   B. The first statement is correct; the second statement is incorrect.
   C. Both statements are incorrect.
   D. The first statement is incorrect; the second statement is correct.

2. Each category in the CDT codes begins with the letter "s" to signify that a service was performed. The second number of the code represents the category and the remaining digits represent the procedure or service.
   A. Both statements are true.
   B. The first statement is true; the second statement is false.
   C. Both statements are false.
   D. The first statement is false; the second statement is true.

3. Define the acronym SMARTER.
   S = _____
   M = _____
   A = _____
   R = _____
   T = _____
   E = _____
   R = _____

4. Select the two most important forms of communication in dentistry.
   1) Writing
   2) Speaking
   3) Listening
   4) Reading
      A. 1 and 2
      B. 1 and 3
      C. 2 and 3
      D. 2 and 4

5. Using BRAN provides the patient with the ability to determine their course of treatment. Select the terms that define the acronym BRAN.
   A. Benefits, rights, accounting options, negotiate
   B. Benefits, risks, alternatives to treatment, no treatment options
   C. Benefits, rights, alternatives to treatment, no treatment options
   D. Benefits, risk, accounting options, no treatment options

6. List three purposes for the Systemized Nomenclature of Dentistry (SNODENT).

   1) _____

   2) _____

   3) _____

7. The most important factor that stands as the foundation of success is:
   A. Goal
   B. Mission
   C. SMART
   D. Vision

8. Which of the following is not a habit of an effective office?
   A. Teams are open to change.
   B. Focused on continuing education to promote lifelong learning.
   C. Profit-focused care.
   D. Superb phone skills and etiquette.

9. All dental professionals have three distinct leadership roles. Which of these is *not* one of these leadership roles?
   A. Leader of self
   B. Leader of the office
   C. Leader of teammates
   D. Leader of patients

Learning Activities

1. Discuss the characteristics of a good leader as outlined in the textbook.

   _____

   _____

   _____

   _____

   _____

   _____

   _____

   _____

   _____

   _____

   _____

   _____

   _____

   _____

   _____

   _____

   _____

2. Refer to the textbook. Choose 3 of the 13 behaviors that leaders and teams embody from the book *Speed of Trust*. Discuss how you will apply these behaviors to your clinical practice.

_____

_____

_____

_____

_____

_____

_____

_____

_____

_____

_____

_____

_____

_____

_____

_____

_____

3. Review the Current Dental Terminology (CDT) codes. Identify the codes for a patient who receives the following treatment: adult prophylaxis, periodic examination, 4BWX. Determine the code for periodontal scaling and root planing for four or more teeth in a quadrant.

_____

_____

_____

_____

_____

_____

_____

_____

_____

_____

_____

_____

_____

_____

_____

_____

_____

Board Style Review Questions

1. An ideal description of what the practice will look like in the short- and long-term defines which of these terms?
   A. Goal
   B. Mission
   C. SMART
   D. Vision

2. All of the following are characteristics of a mission statement *except* for one. Which one is the *exception?*
   A. Should be concise/brief
   B. Should contain nonemotional words
   C. Should state who you are
   D. Should describe what you are about

3. What percentage should dental hygiene retention rates be of the total active patient family?
   A. 50%
   B. 75%
   C. 85%
   D. 95%

4. The direct discussion of financial options is the job of the business team. Clinical team members should focus on the aspects pertaining to clinical matters.
   A. Both statements are correct.
   B. The first statement is correct; the second statement is incorrect.
   C. Both statements are incorrect.
   D. The first statement is incorrect; the second statement is correct.

5. All of the following are major overhead expenses *except* for one. Which one is the *exception?*
   A. Salaries
   B. Business insurance
   C. Dental supplies
   D. Payroll deductions

6. The ideal range for general practice overhead is:
   A. 35% to 45%
   B. 45% to 55%
   C. 55% to 65%
   D. 70% to 75%

7. All of the following are true about CDT *except* for one. Which one is the *exception?*
   A. It is a list of standardized terms and codes.
   B. It was established by the American Dental Association
   C. It is revised approximately every 10 years.
   D. It provides consistency for reporting dental services.

8. A PPO is a preferred provider organization. It is a contract between the patient and the insurance company.
   A. Both statements are true.
   B. The first statement is true; the second statement is false.
   C. Both statements are false.
   D. The first statement is false; the second statement is true.

9. A fee that is determined by the insurance benefit provider from actual submitted fees for specific procedures is:
   A. Customary
   B. Reasonable
   C. Usual
   D. Usual, customary, reasonable

10. The fee that the dentist uses most often for a given dental procedure is:
    A. Customary
    B. Reasonable
    C. Usual
    D. Usual, customary, reasonable

Chapter 53 | Career Development

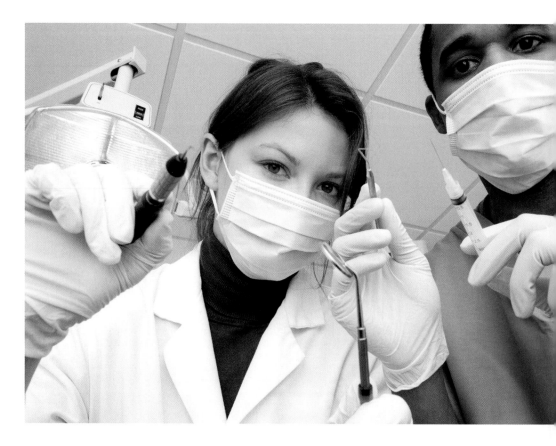

LEARNING OBJECTIVES

After reading this chapter, the student should be able to:

53.1 Describe employment opportunities for a dental hygienist.

53.2 Define the skills needed to find employment.

53.3 Prepare a resume for employment.

53.4 Describe interviewing skills.

53.5 Describe career development strategies.

KEY CONCEPTS

• Dental hygienists should carefully assess employment opportunities available to them.

• Specific skills are necessary to secure employment.

• For a lifetime of job satisfaction, dental hygienists should follow career development strategies.

RELEVANCE TO CLINICAL PRACTICE

Many dental hygienists have been and currently are employed by private dental practices, or, for those with advanced degrees, academic institutions. However, opportunities for employment in school-based clinics, medical practices, and other settings within comprehensive social and health systems networks are also becoming available to dental hygienists. This chapter discusses the skills and strategies needed to secure and maintain employment in a variety of settings.

The Basics

1. List the various employment opportunities for a dental hygienist other than in the dental office setting.

_____   _____

_____   _____

_____   _____

2. Develop a short-term and a long-term career goal.

Short-term goal _____

_____

_____

_____

_____

_____

Long-term goal _____

_____

_____

_____

_____

3. Differentiate between a chronological resume and a functional resume.

_____

_____

_____

_____

_____

_____

4. A curriculum vitae (CV) is:
1) More descriptive than a resume
2) Usually required for academic positions
3) Preferred for most entry-level dental hygiene positions
  A. 1 and 2
  B. 1 and 3
  C. 2 and 3
  D. Only 3

5. What is the first step in career planning?
  A. Assess skills
  B. Advance your education
  C. Set short- and long-term goals
  D. Evaluate career satisfaction

Learning Activities

1. Participate in a mock interview.

2. Prepare a cover letter and resume to review with a mentor.

3. Make a list of skills needed to obtain dental hygiene employment.

Board Style Review Questions

1. Where can the dental hygienist find employment as a health service officer?
  A. United States Public Health Service (USPHS)
  B. National Health Service Corps (NHSC)
  C. Veteran's Affairs (VA) Clinic
  D. Federal prisons

2. Which agency helps to recruit health providers to serve in health professional shortage areas?
  A. United States Public Health Service (USPHS)
  B. National Health Service Corps (NHSC)
  C. Veteran's Affairs (VA) Clinic
  D. Federal prisons

3. Which of these options could provide employment opportunities for the dental hygienist?
1) ADHA website
2) Classified ads in the newspaper
3) Word of mouth through friends or family
4) Government websites
  A. 1 and 2
  B. 1 and 4
  C. 1, 2, and 4
  D. 1, 2, 3, and 4

4. Identify the best method for gaining employment.
  A. Submitting a resume directly to an office.
  B. Participating in a personal interview.
  C. Calling local offices.
  D. Mailing a resume and cover letter.

5. A descriptive, comprehensive format is preferred for a resume. The resume should include credentials, employment history, accomplishments, professional memberships, skills, and community activities.
  A. Both statements are true.
  B. The first statement is true; the second statement is false.
  C. Both statements are false.
  D. The first statement is false; the second statement is true.

6. Choose the best description for chronological resumes.
   A. Emphasizes individual skills
   B. Emphasizes accomplishments
   C. Lists experiences in reverse chronological order
   D. Lists experiences in chronological order

7. The role of the dental hygienist as an advocate is to:
   A. Lobby to change laws
   B. Coordinate clinics
   C. Provide clinical care
   D. Conduct research

8. The traits associated with a health-care professional are all rooted in maleficence. This ethical principle pertains to being trustworthy.
   A. Both statements are correct.
   B. The first statement is correct; the second statement is incorrect.
   C. Both statements are incorrect.
   D. The first statement is incorrect; the second statement is correct.

9. All of the following should be avoided during an interview *except* for one. Which one is the *exception?*
   A. Discussion of marital status
   B. Discussion of appointment length for patients
   C. Chewing gum
   D. Speaking of controversial issues

10. In which of these settings does the hygienist not have an opportunity to work as a U.S. civil service employee?
    A. Veteran's Affairs Clinic
    B. Military base
    C. Federal prison
    D. Dental industry

Chapter 54 | Lifelong Learning

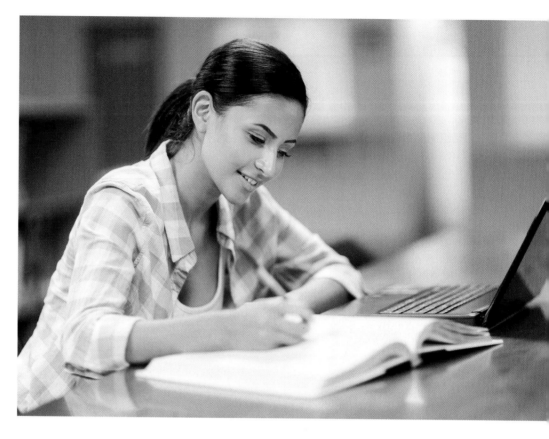

LEARNING OBJECTIVES

After reading this chapter, the student should be able to:

54.1 Define lifelong learning.

54.2 Describe the differences between andragogy and pedagogy.

54.3 Explain critical thinking.

54.4 Define evidence-based practice.

54.5 List various ways in which the Registered Dental Hygienist is able to obtain continuing education after graduation.

54.6 Explain why lifelong learning can be beneficial to both practitioner and patient.

KEY CONCEPTS

• Lifelong learning can help individuals remain current in their discipline.

• Professional responsibility requires the pursuit of continual learning.

• Multiple modalities exist to deliver advanced dental hygiene degrees and continuing education.

• Individual states determine the continuing education criteria for continued licensure.

RELEVANCE TO CLINICAL PRACTICE

The dental hygienist is an integral part of the health-care profession. The dental hygienist sees patients as often as every 3 to 6 months, giving the dental hygienist a unique opportunity to evaluate intraoral and extraoral tissues. Often, the dental hygienist is the first to identify lesions or abnormalities that are associated with systemic disease. As such, it is the dental hygienist's responsibility to stay abreast of new information and modalities in the dental hygiene field by making a commitment to lifelong learning. This chapter discusses the value and effects of lifelong learning for dental hygienists and outlines opportunities for continual study, such as advanced education, continuing education, and self-study.

The Basics

1. Lifelong learning is *best* described as:
   A. Analysis of information, clarification, and evaluation of new knowledge
   B. Teacher-centered
   C. Self-directed, active learning that includes experiential learning
   D. Lifelong and life-wide learning

2. Which of the following *best* describes critical thinking?
   A. Analysis of information, clarification, and evaluation of new knowledge
   B. Teacher-centered
   C. Self-directed, active learning that includes experiential learning
   D. Lifelong and life-wide learning

3. Identify the components of the acronym PICO for composing a well-defined question.

   P =_____

   I =_____

   C =_____

   O =_____

4. To answer questions using evidence-based patient treatment, a dental hygienist must:

   1) _____

   2) _____

   3) _____

5. Order the steps in the evidence-based practice process.

   _____   A. Decide whether evidence is relevant to practice.

   _____   B. Review efficacy of application and improve where necessary.

   _____   C. Compose a well-defined question.

   _____   D. Determine the accuracy of evidence using critical thinking.

   _____   E. Locate credible resources to help answer the question.

6. Be familiar with opportunities to participate in continuing education. List two possible options.
   1) _____ 2) _____

7. List the ideal critical thinking skills.

_____	_____
_____	_____
_____	_____
_____	_____
_____	

Learning Activities

1. In small groups, discuss considerations that relate to advancing the profession of dental hygiene. Present each group's key points to the class.

2. Research the various state labels for direct access, such as collaborative practice, limited access permit, etc. Compare and contrast the scope of practice associated with these credentials.

3. Review the dental hygiene licensing and regulatory agency requirements for the state in which you intend to practice. Note the appropriate continuing education credentials required.

Board Style Review Questions

1. Which of the following organizations developed the Standards for Continuing Education and approves continuing education courses?
   A. AADH
   B. ADEA
   C. ADHA
   D. IFDH

2. Advanced education in dental hygiene includes:
   A. Entry-level degree for clinical practice
   B. Certificate or associate degree specific to clinical dental hygiene
   C. Course of study beyond the level required for clinical practice

3. Professional dental hygiene organizations serve to:
   1) Set policy
   2) Guide member progress
   3) Provide licensure
      A. 1 and 2
      B. 1 and 3
      C. 2 and 3

4. Which organization has a mission "to advance the art and science of dental hygiene and to promote the highest standards of education and practice in the profession"?
   A. American Dental Education Association (ADEA)
   B. American Dental Hygienists' Association (ADHA)
   C. International Federation of Dental Hygienists (IFDH)

5. State requirements for continuing education vary from 6 to 100 hours per licensing period. Licensing periods have renewal periods every 1 or 2 years.
   A. Both statements are true.
   B. The first statement is true; the second is false.
   C. Both statements are false.
   D. The first statement is false; the second is true.

6. In pedagogy, consideration is given to academics and life experiential learning. Andragogy involves the teacher evaluating the learning.
   A. Both statements are true.
   B. The first statement is true; the second is false.
   C. Both statements are false.
   D. The first statement is false; the second is true.

7. In which type of learning do teachers function more like coaches?
    A. Andragogy
    B. Pedagogy
    C. Self-directed learning

8. Health-care professionals are accountable to the public when making treatment decisions; therefore, the dental hygienist must participate as a lifelong learner.
    A. Both the statement and the reason are correct.
    B. The statement is correct; the reason is incorrect.
    C. Both the statement and reason are incorrect.
    D. The statement is incorrect; the reason is correct.

9. Which of the following workforce models does the American Dental Hygienists' Association recommend?
    A. Advanced Dental Hygiene Practitioner (ADHP)
    B. Community Dental Health Coordinator (CDHC)
    C. Dental Health Aide Therapists (DHAT)
    D. Dental Therapist (DT)

Rubrics/Process Evaluations

Process Evaluation Template		
Evidence-Based Decision-Making		
Evaluation Criteria	**Criteria Met? (Y/N)**	**Comments**
Student recognizes the patient's condition.		
Student considers an interaction.		
Student provides a comparison interaction.		
Student acknowledges possible outcomes.		
Student composes a well-defined question using PICO.		
Student locates credible resources to help address the PICO question.		
Student determines the accuracy of evidence using critical thinking skills.		
Student decides if the evidence is relevant to clinical application.		
Student reviews efficacy of application.		
Documentation appropriately noted in treatment notes.		